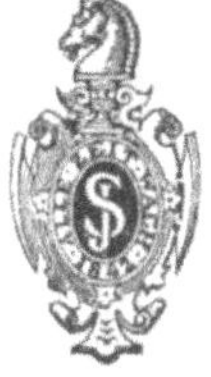

Recent Results in Cancer Research

Fortschritte der Krebsforschung

Progrès dans les recherches sur le cancer

22

Edited by

V. G. Allfrey, New York · M. Allgöwer, Basel · K. H. Bauer, Heidelberg · I. Berenblum, Rehovoth · F. Bergel, Jersey · J. Bernard, Paris · W. Bernhard, Villejuif N. N. Blokhin, Moskva · H. E. Bock, Tübingen · P. Bucalossi, Milano · A. V. Chaklin, Moskva · M. Chorazy, Gliwice · G. J. Cunningham, Richmond · W. Dameshek, Boston M. Dargent, Lyon · G. Della Porta, Milano · P. Denoix, Villejuif · R. Dulbecco, La Jolla · H. Eagle, New York · R. Eker, Oslo · P. Grabar, Paris · H. Hamperl, Bonn R. J. C. Harris, London · E. Hecker, Heidelberg · R. Herbeuval, Nancy · J. Higginson, Lyon · W. C. Hueper, Fort Myers · H. Isliker, Lausanne · D. A. Karnofsky, New York · J. Kieler, København · G. Klein, Stockholm · H. Koprowski, Philadelphia · L. G. Koss, New York · G. Martz, Zürich · G. Mathé, Villejuif · O. Mühlbock, Amsterdam · W. Nakahara, Tokyo · V. R. Potter, Madison · A. B. Sabin, Cincinnati · L. Sachs, Rehovoth · E. A. Saxén, Helsinki · W. Szybalski, Madison H. Tagnon, Bruxelles · R. M. Taylor, Toronto · A. Tissières, Genève · E. Uehlinger, Zürich · R. W. Wissler, Chicago · T. Yoshida, Tokyo

Editor in chief
P. Rentchnick, Genève

Springer-Verlag Berlin · Heidelberg · New York 1969

Tumor Specific Transplantation Antigen

By

Pavel Koldovský

With 19 Figures

Springer-Verlag Berlin · Heidelberg · New York 1969

*Pavel Koldovský, M. D., c/o Wistar Institute,
36, Street at Spruce, Philadelphia, PA 21 / USA*

Sponsored by the Swiss League against Cancer

ISBN-13: 978-3-642-88538-9   e-ISBN-13: 978-3-642-88536-5
DOI: 10.1007/978-3-642-88536-5

Title No. 3637

Softcover reprint of the hardcover 1st edition 1969

Contents

Interest in the immunobiology of tumours is as old as the concept of experimental oncology itself. The past years have witnessed the continnous ebb and flow of this interest and a greater understanding of the entire field has mainly depended on the demonstration of a tumour-specific antigen. Although antigenic differences between normal and tumour tissues have repeatedly been found, it has been felt that some other factors may also be responsible; for example, an inadequate sensitivity of the techniques failing to detect the trace amounts of the same antigen in normal tissues, the possible presence of a necroantigen, etc. Until fairly recently the investigators were extremely sceptical of the existence of tumour antigens, and convincing evidence for the presence of such antigens in human tumours has not as yet been presented.

Specific tumour antigens have been demonstrated in experimental tumours, but it is not known how many types of them may exist. The method of detection is of major importance and it is difficult to say which methods detect distinct antigens and which methods identical antigens. There exist at least two distinct specific antigens: the complement-fixing antigen of the tumours induced by DNA and RNA viruses and the antigen responsible for transplantation resistance. It seems therefore useful to define the method used for the detection of the antigenic differences between the tumour and normal tissues, though, for example, the antigen detected by the adoptive transfer of immunity is probably identical with that responsible for transplantation resistance.

In the very beginning, research in tumour immunology has been developing along two lines — the determination of antigenic differences by serological methods and the possibility of resistance induction on the basis of immunity directed against the tumour. For serological analysis heterologous and allogeneic antisera were used, but it is now very difficult to say whether a specific antigen was involved in those experiments. These methods made it possible to detect the antigen which was specific for the tumour tissues, but was also present in subthreshold amounts in normal tissues (cf. WOGLOM 1929, ZILBER 1957, DAY 1965).

In this review attention will be concentrated on the tumour antigen responsible for transplantation resistance. Resistance has to be induced in an autologous or syngeneic relationships (i. e., within an inbred, antigenically homogeneous, strain of animals from which the tumour originated). The antigen involved will then be present only in tumour cells and will be important for the viability of cells so that immunity to it will bring about the destruction of cells. Furthermore, the antigen will be present not only in some tumour cells, but in all tumour cells so that the whole tumour may be destroyed. SJÖGREN (1964) proposed to designate this antigen as tumour specific transplantation antigen (TSTA). Such an antigen is therefore capable of inducing a state which can be defined as autoimmune disease of the tumour, and is thus to some extent comparable, to an organ-specific antigen.

It may be useful to show how the views on this antigen have developed. The initial experiments carried out at the turn of the century have shown that the animal that had rejected a tumour transplant was resistant to subsequent challenge with the same tumour. Although resistance was shown to be associated with the immune mechanisms, specific antitumour immunity was not involved. In these experiments the tumours transplanted between members of an antigenically non-homogeneous population or even between different strains. It was demonstrated that immunity was directed against normal transplantation antigens present in the tumour tissue. The antigenic composition of normal transplantation antigens in the tumours is identical with that in normal tissues and is governed by the same genetic laws (LITTLE and TYZZER, 1916).

It has been stressed in the definition of TSTA that immune resistance has to be induced in an autologous relationship or within an inbred strain of animals. The first inbred strains of mice have been established in 1901, but the first attempt to induce immunity against a spontaneous tumour indigenous to an inbred mouse strain has presumably been made by LUMSDEN in the late 1920's or early 1930's (LUMSDEN, 1931). The author used the inbred strain of Lashop Loeb from Buffalo, which was in its 32nd and further generations at the time of the experiment, and the tumour that arose spontaneously in this strain. However, evidence concerning the existence of a tumour-specific antigen was not satisfactory because only 3 out of 170 mice were resistant, and both residual heterozygosity and mutation in transplantation antigens could be suspected in the mice used. Nevertheless, LUMSDEN must be credited with having drawn attention to the possibility of using the experimental model that has been extensively studied some twenty-five years later.

CLOWES (1905) observed that spontaneous tumour regression leads to the regression of a further inoculum of the same tumour while transplantability is still very high in control animals. His observation stimulated BESREDKA and GROSS (1935) to carry out experiments on the induction of tumour regression in mice and to study its effect on the fate of a subsequent transplant of the same tumour. The latter authors found that after the intradermal inoculation of a small, precisely defined, amount of a tumour cell suspension the tumours began to grow, but then "spontaneously" regressed presumably as a result of insufficient metabolic exchange during their rapid growth. After the tumour had regressed, the mice were also resistant to a subcutaneous inoculation of the same tumour. Since both CLOWES's observation and BESREDKA and GROSS's experiments were carried out with genetically (antigenically) non-homogeneous strains of mice, the resistance obtained might have been due to immunity against transplantation individual-specific rather than tumour-specific antigens of the tumours used.

A few years later, the same method was applied by GROSS to inbred mice and methylcholanthrene-induced tumours indigenous to this strain (1943 a, b). The author used the C3H strain, which has been maintained by brother x sister mating for more than 20 years at the time of the experiment. Of the 112 mice inoculated intra-dermally with 0.01 ml of a 20% tumour cell suspension, 91 mice died with progressively growing tumours, but 21 mice showed regression of tumours after initial growth. These and a control group of untreated mice were challenged with 0.01—0.03 ml of a 20% tumour cell suspension. While all the controls died with progressively growing tumours, no tumours grew in experimental animals, or the tumours began to grow and then regressed. The TSTA has thus been demonstrated in methylcholanthrene-induced tumours, but some critical objections were raised which will be discussed later. Gross pointed to an interesting fact that immunity against carcinogenic tumours had no influence on the appearance of spontaneous tumours. A further GROSS's finding relative to the size of the immunizing and challenge dose was of much importance for studies on TSTA. A large challenge dose has been found to overcome immunity; this finding has been repeatedly confirmed for the antigenic differences of varying strength in the tumour-immune host relationship. It should be mentioned that a similar finding was made by LUMSDEN although his interpretation was not correct. In certain combinations of animals preimmunized with homologous (allogeneic) tumour cells and then challenged with a tumour the "virulence" of which was attenuated by formalin, a difference between the immunized and control group was revealed, but not with a fully "virulent" tumour.

Methods of Induction of Antitumour Immunity

A. Immunization with Viable Tumour Cells

Theoretically, the tumour can grow out of a single cell capable of mitosis. In fact, it was possible to demonstrate growth of the tumour after transplantation of a very small number of tumour cells, also with such heterogeneous tumours as the Walker 256 carcinoma. (However, such tumours transplanted to a variety of animals may be the tumours that are highly adapted and antigenically simple.)

To ensure tumour growth in 100% of control animals, several tens up to ten thousands of tumour cells are usually required. The state of malignancy, that we try to describe as virulence, progressive growth, and also the degree of dedifferentiation of the tumour are of decisive importance. The possible antigenic differences between tumour and host may be important, too. The greater the antigenic difference, the larger the initial inoculum of tumour is necessary. It takes some time before immunity against the tumour develops; if the initial inoculum is sufficiently large so that the rate of tumour growth is more rapid than that of immunity development, the tumour grows progressively until the death of the host. In contrast, if the initial inoculum is small, immunity develops more rapidly and the tumour regresses. Numerous direct and indirect observations indicated that the inoculation itself of viable tumour cells into intact recipients leads to development of immunity. During serial passages the antigenicity of the tumour decreases, and this is accompanied by a decrease in the number of cells needed for successful transfer. Irradiation of the recipient with X-rays results in diminution up to suppression of the host defense mechanisms, and also in reduction of the minimal inoculum. On the other hand, non-specific stimulation of immunity may increase the size of the minimal inoculum.

The use of subthreshold doses seems to be the relatively simplest method of immunization against a syngeneic tumour. Animals, in which the subthreshold dose

1*

of cells does not grow, are usually immunized at the same time; then even the threshold dose fails to grow in them. On increasing the dose gradually, a relatively strong degree of immunity is attained.

PRINCE et al. (1957) found that after an intravenous administration complete immunity was obtained before the implant metastases developed. The animals injected by the intravenous route showed a degree of resistance to the tumour which was inoculated subcutaneously three weeks later.

Another example of immunization with a subminimal dose of cells is immunization with an oncogenic virus (insofar as it is proved that anti-viral immunity is different from antitumour immunity), as has been shown, for example, with polyoma virus (SJÖGREN, 1962). As will be seen in the section on TSTA in relation to aetiology, oncogenic viruses may induce malignat transformation of cells and at the same time the TSTA. If malignant transformation takes place in immunologically mature hosts, the TSTA is recognized as a foreign, distinct antigen, the tumour is rejected as a consequence of immunological reaction of the transplantation type and the resultant state is transplantation resistance against subsequent challenge with tumour cells of the same origin. On the other hand, in newborn animals, malignant transformation and the appearance of cells with a new antigen may lead to a state of immunological tolerance or at least depressed reactivity whereby tumour progression is facilitated.

Another method of immunization with viable tumour tissues makes use of the fact that tumours induced by the same oncogenic virus possess the same tumour-specific antigen. Mice of an inbred strain (e. g., A strain) are injected with the tumour produced in another strain (e. g., C3H). A polyoma tumour, strain-specific for the C3H strain of mice, conceivably regresses in the A strain mice as a result of the difference in normal transplantation antigens. At the same time, mice of the A strain are immunized against the TSTA of the polyoma tumours and are then also resistant to the A strain tumour induced by polyoma virus.

FOLEY (1952) in his experiments started from the finding that a growing tumour is, without any further treatment, capable of immunizing the animals. The difficulty was a safe removal of growing tumours before immunity could be tested. FOLEY therefore inoculated the tumour gradually between the sheets of the auricle and subcutaneously into the tail. The tumour was then completely removed by amputating the auricle or the tail together with some healthy tissue. The tumour grew in the host for several weeks and a continous supply of antigen in small doses appeared to be a very effective method of immunization against a weak antigen.

The difference between GROSS's and BESREDKA's method of immunization as described earlier in this text and the use of subminimal doses is that inadequate nutritional conditions during intracutaneous growth make it possible to use a relatively large inoculum of living cells. Despite this, tumour regression occurred in a comparatively small number of animals (about 20% of animals in GROSS's syngeneic system). This form of immunization is therefore not practical. Nevertheless, a modification based on the ligature of subcutaneously (BALDWIN, 1955) or intracutaneously (KOLDOVSKY 1961 a) growing tumours is one of the most effective methods of immunization.

With leukaemia L1210, which is very sensitive to amethopterin, resistance to subsequent inoculum of the same leukaemia (GOLDIN, 1960) was observed in mice that had been cured with this chemotherapeutic agent. The result suggests that the therapeutic value of cytostatics should also be considered from the immunological aspects.

GORER'S experiments (GORER et al., 1962) on the effect of allogeneic serum against the X antigen of some leukaemias showed that insofar as complete regression of leukaemia occurs, the resultant state is again transplantation resistance.

An unusual procedure of immunization was used by GOLDNER et al. (1959) against a spontaneous ascites tumour 9a which arose in inbred rats. The antigenic homogeneity of the strain used was controlled by skin grafts. The tumour killed 100% of the recipients when injected intraperitoneally. Subcutaneously injected tumour regressed and thereafter immunity was present even against an intraperitoneal application. This unexpected behaviour of the tumour is in agreement with the results obtained with heterotopic (subcutaneous) transplants of autologous tumour tissues carried out by SOUTHAM and his colleagues (SOUTHAM, 1965) in humans.

B. Immunization with Tumour after Eliminating its Capacity for Repopulation

With this method, immunization does not carry the possible hazard of producing distant metastases which may develop following each inoculation of live tumour cells. It is only difficult to find the way of preventing growth of the tumour tissues and of producing the slightest damage to the tumour antigen.

In the allogeneic relationship against normal transplantation antigens, immunization with heat-killed (FLEXNER JOBLING, 1910), frozen (CASEY, 1949), or lyophilized tumour cells (KALISS, 1965) generally leads to a reverse paradoxical phenomenon—the tumour growth is facilitated in interstrain combinations. In the syngeneic relationship, immunization with lyophilized tumour using FREUND'S adjuvant results, on the contrary, in transplantation resistance (FINK et al., 1953).

The finding that the regressing tumour can induce a strong state of immunity instigated attempts to immunize with necrotic material. Some degree of immunity was obtained with a, formalin-treated tumour (LUMSDEN, 1931). Since the antigenic homogeneity of the animals used was not ensured, immunity to normal transplantation antigens might have been involved. The use of necrotic material after the ligature of a subcutaneously growing tumour revealed strong antigenicity of this material. In experiments with carcinogen-induced tumours in inbred rats LEWIS and APTEKMAN (1951) demonstrated a stronger antigenicity of the tissue in which atrophy took longer, and the ligature was removed later. While immunization with tissue, which had been ligatured for two days, produced resistance in only 70% of the animals, the tissue undergoing atrophy for 4 days led to resistance in 100% of the animals.

However, the use of killed cells not fully remove the danger of inducing enhancement (see Enhancement against TSTA). MIROFF et al. (1955) found that the tumour ZBC heated to 70° C for an hour and injected into Z(C3H) mice accelerated the growth of a subsequent tumour inoculum. (Neither in this experiment nor in the next one was it analysed whether immunological enhancement was in fact involved.) Similarly, PRINCE et al. (1957) found that drB carcinoma inoculated subcutaneously into DBA/1 mice after previous autolysis for 24 hrs at 37.5° C caused an accelerated growth of the second tumour implant. The authors studied the influence of varying lengths of incubation of tumour cells at this temperature on their immunizing capacity, and at the same time followed the immunizing potency of tumour tissue cut to pieces 1—2 cm in size. This tissue was diluted 1:1,500 and the suspension was injected intravenously in amounts of 0.05 ml. Test inoculation was performed 4 and 18 days after immunization with autolysed tumour and 17—19 days after immunization with alcohol-killed tumour. While the tumour incubated for 1—5 hrs at 37.5° C elicited resistance, the material incubated for a longer period of time led to an accelerated growth. On the other hand, alcohol-killed tumour cells induced the state of transplantation resistance in the same experimental system.

FINK (1953) obtained transplantation resistance after the inoculation of BALB/c mice with lyophilized methylcholanthrene-induced tumour (S62L) incorporated in FREUND's adjuvant; without adjuvant this was not achieved.

Although large doses of irradiation are capable of influencing the antigenicity of serum proteins (WANG LING FANG, 1960), immunization with tumour suspensions irradiated with 14,000—20,000 R is very effective against tumours induced by chemical carcinogens (REVESZ, 1960). However, the TSTA of polyoma tumours may lose its immunogenicity after doses of 8,000 R (SJÖGREN, 1962) and the TSTA of mouse RSV-induced tumours is also severly damaged by irradiation doses higher than 10,000 R (BUBENIK et al., 1965).

No loss of antigenicity was observed in tumour cells whose capacity for re-population was arrested by cytostatics in vitro.

The possibility of immunizing with subcellular fractions or biochemically defined tumour tissue components will be discussed in the section on the Characteristics of TSTA.

Methods of Detection of Antitumour Immunity

It is well known that a too high challenge dose can overcome immunity so that it is impossible to find any difference between the control and immunized groups. Hence the so-called minimal dose must be determined for each tumour, i. e. the amount of viable tumour cells capable of growing in 100% of the control animals using a standard method of inoculation. This minimal dose shows great variations for different tumours and is influenced not only by the antigenicity of the tumour used, but also by its general biological properties. The degree of immunity achieved for different tumours is therefore best determined not by comparing the absolute number of cells overcoming immunity, but by the number of the minimal doses.

Immunity directed against the tumour antigen, as against every weak antigen, develops very slowly. Thus, testing performed e. g. on day 10 after immunization (this time is sufficient for development of immunity to transplantation antigens controlled by the H-2 locus) does not usually detect any, or very weak, antitumour immunity, whereas by day 30 a large percentage of immunized animals may already be resistant.

Immunity is most easily detected when a significant number of immunized animals are resistant, whereas the tumour grows in 100% of the controls. Such an ideal situation is rarely encountered and consequently more sensitive methods must be used. Most frequently, the tumours in experimental and control groups are measured in three (or two) directions perpendicular to one another and the growth curves of individual tumours or of the mean values for separate groups are constructed. This method is very sensitive and can detect very weak immunity which is manifest only in the initial phases of tumour growth and may be later obliterated by progressive tumour growth. A less sensitive modification of this method is comparison of tumour growth rates on the basis of survival times of animals in separate groups.

Regional lymph nodes and spleen react to the stimulation with a tumour antigen by proliferation detectable by simple measurement (weighing) of these organs, or microscopically (WOODRUFF and SYMES, 1962). However, this reaction is a less accurate method of detection — it needs not at all be induced by a weak antigen, or may be strong when a secondary (bacterial) infection is present. Nevertheless, if regional lymph node cells or spleen cells are used for adoptive transfer of immunity against the tumour, then the reaction of transplantation type against the tumour antigen can be quite accurately detected.

Cells of malignant lymphomas form nodules in the spleen when applied intravenously. The number of nodules in a certain range depends upon the number of injected cells. Moreover, the state of immunity in the animal is of decisive importance — less nodules are formed in immune animals and conversely, more nodules in animals with reduced reactivity (AXELRAD, 1965). The same is probably true of the number of the lung metastases in solid tumours (carcinomas, sarcomas) when their cells are inoculated intravenously.

GRAFFI et al. (1962) suggested that an intravenous injection of a trypsinized tumour cell suspension and comparison of the number of metastases in the lung tissues and in the organs of the body circulation in the control and immunized group was a very sensitive method of detecting antitumour immunity.

The amount of tumour antigen can also be determined, but only in relation to other tumours. In the first place, this is performed by comparing the capacity of equally large amounts of tumour tissue with abolished repopulating ability to induce a similar degree of resistance. The degree of resistance can be relatively accurately expressed as the number of minimal doses of tumour cells capable of overcoming it. The state of immunity can also be estimated by the proportion of immune and tumour cells in adoptive transfer. Finally, in the tumours showing good cytotoxic reactions with syngeneic serum, the amount of antigen can be determined in certain material by its capacity to absorb the cytotoxic activity of a standard antiserum. HOUGHTON (1965) modified WIGZELL's method of detecting cytotoxicity by means of the release of labelled chromium (^{51}Cr) for Moloney lymphoma. He absorbed thes serum of known activity with the material tested and assayed its antigenicity from the degree of absorption.

In detecting TSTA by means of the transplantation test on a living animal, it should be borne in mind that non-specific stimulation may also stimulate a specific immune response, especially when the challenge dose is close to the minimal dose. The recipients are therefore irradiated with 350 r (for mice) 24 hours before the challenge dose. This irradiation dose removes the primary response, but the secondary response is not considerably decreased. However, a weak secondary response can be practically abolished by irradiation. The test for specificity by means of adoptive transfer of immunity requires various proportions of immune and control cells to be used, and with this titration the test is relatively reliable. The best method is the use of control immune cells from non-specifically stimulated animals. The simplest test of specificity of the observed transplantation reaction against the tumour is an adequate non-specific stimulation of control animals.

Tumour-Specificity of the Antigen Detected by the Method of Transplantation Resistance

Immunity directed against a tumour induced within an inbred strain and shortly passaged has been demonstrated as early as in 1940's. However, the question remained whether this immunity could be attributed to a tumour-specific antigen, or to residual heterozygosity in antigenicity of the particular inbred strain or of the tumour employed (or the donor of the primary tumour). Moreover, mutations in transplantation antigens within inbred strains of mice have been observed. As a rule, the antigenic homogeneity is tested among only some individuals of the breeding nucleus, or among individuals randomly selected from the population already produced for the experiment. Control experiments were therefore carried out to demonstrate the tumour-specificity of TSTA. PREHN and MAIN immunized one group of mice with the tumour, and another one with normal tissues from the tumour donor. Animals preimmunized with the tumour were resistant to challenge with their own tumour, while those preimmunized with normal tissues showed a similar tumour growth as the controls. Attempts to immunize with the tumour against normal tissues also confirmed the specificity of TSTA. Convincing evidence was provided by KLEIN et al. (1960), who demonstrated that immunity against the tumour could be induced even in animals in which the tumour originally arose. They inoculated methyl-cholanthrene into the thigh muscles and when a tumour appeared the limb was amputated. Thus, they could test immunity against really autologous tumours. Testing by means of skin grafts controlling the antigenic homogeneity of the mice used is more complicated (KOLDOVSKÝ, 1961 a). This method, however, made it possible to test the specificity of spontaneous tumours. The skin grafts were gradually exchanged between mice of two strains (A and CBA) — males and females. The mouse No. 2. received a graft from mouse No. 1 and No. 3, mouse No. 4 from No. 2 and 4, and in this way, continuous chains were formed ensuring the antigenic homogeneity of all mice in the particular chain. With spontaneous adenocarcinomas of the females, it was only a matter of time before the tumour arose in a mouse, some of the males were injected with methylcholanthrene. Furthermore, the skin grafts were transferred from this "tumour conferring group" to a group of mice which were later immunized. Permanent acceptance of the grafts was evidence that the donor group did not possess any antigen which would not be shared by the immunized group. A degree of transplantation resistance was revealed in each tumour and thus the tumour specificity of acquired immunity was also confirmed by this experiment.

In tumours induced by oncogenic viruses, the tumour antigen is common to all tumours induced by a particular oncogenic virus. The same applies to the interspecies relationships. It is unlikely that this antigen might occur by mutation and would have nothing to do with the malignant process. This antigen appears to be the direct product of the genetic information carried by the virus into the cell.

Specific Tumour Antigenicity and the Aetiology of the Tumour Chemical Carcinogens

Some of the experiments in which resistance against carcinogen-induced tumours and hence the presence of TSTA have been demonstrated were referred to in the previous section. Such tumours possess a relatively strong tumour-specific antigen. Three carcinogenic chemicals are now known to induce tumours that contain a tumour-specific antigen. These are methylcholanthrene (GROSS 1943, PREHN and MAIN 1957), benzpyrene (KOLDOVSKÝ, 1961 a; OLD, BOYSE, 1962; GLOBERSON and FELDMAN, 1964) and dibenzanthrancene (KOLDOVSKÝ, 1961 a; PREHN, 1960 a). The fourth substance—urethane—considerably different in its chemical structure was studied by PREHN, who found that only one out of seven lung adenocarcinomas induced by urethane was antigenic under the given experimental conditions. The importance of the method of induction for the occurrence of a tumour antigen was confirmed by PREHN and MAIN (1957) showing that spontaneous fibrosarcomas histologically indistinguishable from fibrosarcomas induced by methylcholanthrene did not contain any tumour antigen. Carcinogen-induced leukaemias such as leukaemia L1210 also contains the TSTA.

Of particular interest are the experiments of GORER and AMOS (1956) and GORER et al. (1962) with EL 4 leukaemia and other leukaemias induced by chemical carcinogens. They demonstrated the presence of the so-called X-antigen in these leukaemias by means of in vivo cytotoxic activity of allogeneic antiserum absorbed in vivo. The leukaemias wer induced by di-benzanthracene, with the exception of CL2 leukaemia, which arose by the intracerebral injection of methylcholanthrene. It was interesting that spontaneous leukaemias CL3 and EL6 possessed the same specific antigen. In a more detailed analysis, GORER et al. (1962) revealed the existence of at least three types of X antigen represented in leukaemias EL4, EL6, EL8. The EL4 type was also present in EL5, EL7 and EL7b leukaemias, but the antigen EL5 did not cross-react with antigen EL7b. GORER therefore assumed that antigen EL4 was composed of at least two types of antigen which corresponded to EL5 and EL7b.

OLD et al. (1962) studied the tumours induced by methyl-cholanthrene and benzpyrene in inbred mice. Numerous factors are capable of influencing the incidence of tumours after the injection of carcinogenic agents. They demonstrated that similar factors might play a role in the induction or expression of a tumour-specific antigen. Males are more sensitive to the threshold doses of methylcholanthrene than females. No such difference has been observed with benzpyrene, which as a carcinogen is more effective in inducing the tumours than methylcholanthrene. Most of the benzpyrene-induced tumours are less antigenic than tumours induced by methyl-cholanthrene. OLD presumed that the difference in cancerogenic capacity was the reason why benzpyrene-induced tumours were less antigenic. In regard to the differences in antigenicity and in sex, detectable only for methylcholanthrene, the finding should be recalled that females are immunologically more reactive against transplantation antigens than males (BATCHELOR, 1965).

PREHN found that not only sarcomas induced by methylcholanthrene, but also mouse mammary carcinomas induced in the same manner, were antigenic. However, the so-called spontaneous mammary carcinomas do not generally elicit immune response (PREHN, 1965). The carcinogenic origin of skin carcinomas (PASTERNAK et al., 1964) is of equal importance for their antigenicity.

Virus-Induced Tumours

The question of genuinely antiviral immunity will not be discussed here as it does not involve immunity against tumour tissue itself, but a neutralizing action against oncogenic viruses (cf. GORER, 1961).

The TSTA has been demonstrated practically for all tumours induced by oncogenic viruses insofar as specific transplantation antitumour immunity has been studied. The first virus-dependent TSTA detected in tumours induced by SE-polyoma virus has been most extensively studied in this respect.

In their initial work HABEL and ATANASIU (1959) did not find any difference in the growth of a polyoma virus-induced tumour in hamsters preimmunized with the virus and the control hamsters. However, they did find resistance in mice (HABEL, 1961). SJÖGREN et al. (1961) and SJÖGREN and RINGERTZ (1962) obtained passageable tumours in mice and performed detailed studies. They tested 15 transplantable, polyoma-induced tumours and two spontaneous mammary carcinomas with regard to their capacity to grow in 3 groups of mice: 1. untreated control group. 2. group preimmunized with the virus (supernatant from tissue cultures), 3. group preimmunized with heavily irradiated tumour cells. Immunity against 11 tumours was tested by means of a minimal inoculum. Of these tumours, seven did not all grow in mice preimmunized with the virus, three grew in some animals and only one showed no difference when compared with the controls. In the group preimmunized with irradiated cells against two tumours, some degree of resistance was observed and a weak enhancing effect on two other tumours was noted. The control tumours — spontaneous mammary carcinomas — grew equally well in both control and preimmunized groups. Later on, SJÖGREN studied this question in detail in a series of experiments (1962, 1964 a, b, c). He demonstrated the specificity of the particular reaction since preirradiation of immunized mice with a total-body dose of 400 R had no influence on the result of the experiment — the mice remained resistant. The lymphoid cells and serum from virus-preimmunized mice inhibited the growth of a syngeneic tumour graft. It is also possible to preimmunize the animals with an allogeneic tumour against a syngeneic tumour. Hence the antigen involved is common to all the tumours induced by polyoma virus. Theoretically, either actually the virus, or a new cellular surface antigen induced by the virus might have been involved. Since immunization with a tumour not containing the virus is also possible, and resistance had been proved even in animals possessing no antiviral antibodies, and the immunity obtained by inactivated virus had no effect on the fate of subsequent tumour graft, SJÖGREN concluded that immunity was directed against the TSTA induced. This antigen has also been shown to cross-react in the inter-specific relationships (HABEL, 1963).

The most feasible explanation of the mechanism of antitumour immunity induced by immunization with a virus-containing supernatant (cell-free supernatant) is that even in adult mice the polyoma virus causes malignant transformation of cells and at the same time induces the TSTA in them. The cells are recognized as foreign and are destroyed by the transplantation reaction.

Similarly, transplantation resistance against Moloney lymphoma was proved in mice preimmunized with Moloney virus. Again, the antigen involved was common to all tumours induced by this virus and did not cross-react with tumours of other aetiology (SACHS, 1962; KLEIN, 1964).

A very weak TSTA was also detected in tumours induced by SV40 virus (KOCH and SABIN, 1963). The antigen was specific for this virus and KHERRA et al. (1963) found that resistance was directed against a new cellular antigen but not against the virus.

In tumours induced by Gross virus resistance was detected after preimmunization with subminimal doses or after immunization with allogeneic tumour of the same origin (KLEIN et al., 1962).

PATERNAK demonstrated the possibility of obtaining resistance against tumours induced by Graffi virus after preimmunization of rats with subminimal doses or with heavily irradiated cells. Preimmunization against heterologous rat tumour of the same origin using a cell-free filtrate from the mouse Graffi lymphoma led to immunity. No cross-reaction against the Gross antigen was revealed (PASTERNAK, in press).

OLD et al. (1963) published a comparative study on specific antigens of mouse leukaemias induced by oncogenic viruses. According to the method of detection they distinguish at least three antigens — antigen responsible for transplantation resistance, antigen detectable by fluorescent antibodies and CF antigen. As a rule, the antigens are strictly specific for a particular group of leukaemias. According to the way, in which individual leukaemias cross-react with TSTA, they fall into four antigenic groups: G (Gross virus), FMR (Friend, Moloney, Rauscher viruses), TL (thymus leukaemic) and E (X antigen in GORER's terminology). In the first two groups the cross-reactions take place not only between the leukaemic cells, but also between the viruses (FINK and RAUCHSCHER, 1964). TL antigen apart from certain leukaemias is also present in the normal thymus of some mouse strains. The last E antigen (GORER et al., 1962) is detectable by allogeneic sera in various leukaemias of carcinogenic and spontaneous origin.

Studies on rabbit papilloma of viral origin showed that this virus may also induce a new cellular antigen. EVANS et al. (1966) found that Shope papilloma regressed after the administration of allogeneic or autologous tissue vaccines. The percentage of regression in vaccinated animals was two to three times that in the controls. KIDD (1938) showed in his experiments that virus neutralizing antibodies had no effect on tumour growth. EVANS (1966) demonstrated that serum from rabbits in which the tumour had regressed, did not influence regression after passive transfer. Since the ability of rabbits to destroy the tumour is not associated with the presence of neutralizing antibodies, it seemed likely that a cellular antigen induced by the virus rather than viral surface antigen responsible for immunity directed against a tumour graft was involved.

Furthermore, EVANS showed that preimmunization with a vaccine prepared from Shope papilloma reduced the take of Vx7 carcinoma by 50%. Vx7 carcinoma is a transplantable tumour which arises by malignant transformation of a papilloma and contains a virus-induced antigen after as many as 100 passages.

The TSTA has also been demonstrated in tumours induced by an avian oncogenic virus — the Rous sarcoma virus in mammals. Of the various strains of Rous virus that are at present being studied, the SCHMIDT-RUPPIN strain seems to be the most malignant for mammals; it induces a relatively high percentage of tumours in mice, rats, guinea-pigs, hamsters, rabbits and monkeys (AHLSTRÖM, 1964). Transplantation immunity against a syngeneic tumour has been successfully induced in both mice (JONSSON, 1964; SJÖGREN, KOLDOVSKÝ, BUBENIK, 1965) and inbred rats (HARRIS, 1967). This immunity can be induced by the subminimal doses of cells and by allogeneic tumours of the same origin. If heavily irradiated cells are used for immunization, the irradiation dose should not be greater than 10,000 R; the dose of 20,000 R reduces the antigenicity so that the irradiated tissue is not effective in inducing immunity (BUBENIK et al., 1965). Immunization with purified virus also leads to immunity (KOLDOVSKÝ et al., 1965; RADZIKHOVSKAYA, 1966); the virus is highly effective especially when the chicken tumour is injected into newborn animals whereby the virus can be released and immunizes for relatively long periods of time (JONSSON, SJÖGREN, 1966). The tumours induced in rats and mice have been found to give weak, but specific cross-reactions (JONSSON, 1966).

Experiments on ducks (SVOBODA, 1961) and turkeys (HARRIS, 1961) reveal that the induction of immunological tolerance to normal chicken tissues facilitates the induction of RSV tumour formation in these animal species after they have achieved immunological maturity. The duck or turkey Rous sarcoma cells are presumed to contain some of normal antigens of the chicken cell. The antigenic alteration, if it occurs at all, is brought about by Rous virus. It would be interesting to find out whether a similar antigenic change, i. e., the presence of a normal chicken antigen, occurs on the cell of a mouse Rous sarcoma. The first experiments along this line provided positive results when the tissues from White Leghorns were used. The specificity of the reaction was confirmed by adoptive transfers. Non-specific stimulation with duck tissues was without any effect (KOLDOVSKÝ et al., 1966). The normal chicken tissues may contain viruses related to RSV (e. g. RAV, RIF), but it is not known whether these may be used for immunization against RSV mouse tumours. Some positive results were obtained in this respect (to be published). Finally, positive, but less obvious results were obtained when tissues from RIF-free Brown Leghorn chickens were used for immunization (KOLDOVSKÝ, 1966). On the other hand, JONSSON and SJÖGREN (1965) observed only non-specific stimulation when using normal chicken tissues. This reaction was removed by preirradiating the mice prior to test inoculation. An equally non-specific stimulation in their experiments was immunization with chicken Rous sarcoma when adult mice were immunized. Later on, they found that immunization of newborn mice with chicken Rous sarcoma led to immunity (1966) when no tumour developed. They explained it by a more intensive and longer stimulation with a specific antigen as the virus is released for longer periods of time and longer transforms the cells in newborn animals. Why should the immunization with tumour lead to only non-specific stimulation in adult animals when a weak, specific immunity may be involved. Likewise, weak (or non-specific) immunity has been detected after immunization with normal chicken tissues. This important question, that is, the "transfer" of antigen by the virus between various species, cannot be answered satisfactorily unless further experiments are done.

Cross-reactions were proved among tumours induced by different variants of Rous virus. Cross-reactions were observed with TSTA of the SCHMIDT-RUPPIN, Prague, BRYAN and HARRIS strain of Rous virus (BUBENÍK, BAUER, 1967).

Immunity Directed against Spontaneous Tumours

Most of the so-called spontaneous tumours in mice are presumably of viral origin. All the tumours induced by the known oncogenic viruses have been proved to contain a TSTA. Despite this, the question of antigenic specificity of spontaneous tumours is still open and the results obtained are contradictory. It is generally difficult to obtain a clear transplantation immunity against these tumours. The unusual behaviour of the spontaneous rat ascites tumour 9a has been referred to in the section on the method of induction of antitumour immunity. HAUSCHKA (1952) in his review on antitumour immunity comes to the conclusion that it is impossible to obtain immunity against the tumours which arise spontaneously within inbred strains. REVESZ (1960) failed to induce immunity against spontaneous tumours although he obtained resistance to carcinogen-induced tumours using the same method in the same mouse strains. The difference between spontaneous and carcinogen-induced tumours has been observed by other authors, too. REVESZ believes that spontaneous tumours do not contain the TSTA, and if such an antigen has been disclosed, this might have been the antigen which arose e. g. by mutation during passages of the tumour, and not the tumour-specific antigen.

HIRSCH et al. (1958) in their studies on antigenicity of spontaneous mammary adenocarcinomas used the inbred C strain of mice (Bagg Albino) between its 69th and 71st generation, and the tumour developed in a mouse from the 69th generation. The tumour from the first passage was used for immunization and from the second passage for testing immunity. Immunization was performed by serial inoculation of viable tumour cells into the auricles and the tail and by the surgical removal of the tumour after initial growth. The difference in survival times between the control and experimental group was statistically significant. The mice in the immunized group survived for an average of 124 days, whereas those in the control group for only 91 days. Similar results were obtained in our laboratory (KOLDOVSKÝ, 1961); immunization by ligature of an intracutaneously growing tumour repeated 6 times led to a significantly prolonged survival of experimental animals as compared to the controls. The reduction of test inoculation dose to 10^2 to 10^3 also failed to detect resistant animals (unpublished results).

On the other hand, MARTINEZ et al. (1958) showed that back-cross mice of the C3H(Z) strain could be immunized with a spontaneous tumour C3H(Z), and a high percentage of these mice were resistant to this tumour — 5% of takes in the experimental group as compared with 90% in the controls. The tumour was at its 53rd passage and thus, REVESZ' objection regarding antigenic mutations during passages cannot be excluded. The model used is in agreement with the laws of inheritance of transplantation antigens and the back-cross hybrids cannot react against antigens of the parental strain, but after the findings of CUDKOWICZ (1961) were published, it is not certain whether this contention can be accepted without any reservation.

PRINCE et al. (1957) reported of another case of resistance to spontaneous tumours. However, even in this case, a long-passaged tumour was involved. Taking into account the possible antigenic mutations it should be remembered that the authors had failed to induce resistance with the same tumour in their earlier experiment (1953).

The failure to induce resistance may be primarily attributed to the absence of tumour antigen of the transplantation type. However, there may be at least two reasons why the detection of resistance fails even if the tumour antigen is present on tumour cells. First, the cause may be the immunoresistance of tumour cells; its mechanism is not yet clear, but the decrease in the number of antigenic receptors on the cell surface may probably play a role. Second, the inability of the recipients to react, in general or in the sense of resistance against the particular tumour antigen. These possibilities will be discussed in the next section, but in connection with spontaneous tumours, the experiments of WEISS et al. (1964) and of ATTIA et al. (1965) should be briefly referred to. These authors found that resistance to spontaneous tumours could be induced in mice genetically identical with the tumour donor, but lacking natural tolerance.

Immunity Directed against Tumours of Various Origin

Experimental tumours have been relatively frequently induced by irradiation, and the methods of their induction (they are mostly leukaemias) have been elaborated. Also from the practical point of view, it is important to know whether these tumours may contain the TSTA. A variety of tumours, even in man, can be induced by irradiation (sunshine, skin carcinoma of the radiologists etc.). In a radiation-induced leukaemia in the CBA strain KOLDOVSKÝ (1962) did not detect any immunity against this leukaemia. Analogous results were obtained by SACHS (1962) in his experiments on radiation-induced leukaemia in the C57BL strain. On the other hand, PASTERNAK et al. (1964) described resistance to tumours induced by UV irradiation. Similarly, NILSSON and REVESZ (In SJÖGREN's review 1965) observed the antigenicity of tumours induced by ^{90}Sr.

KLEIN et al. (1963) studied the antigenicity of tumours induced by cellophane film. The histological structure of tumours induced in this manner is similar to that of tumours induced by chemical carcinogens. However, control experiments revealed that in this case another mechanism of carcinogenesis must have been involved. The powder prepared from the same material or a cellophane film, which is perforated and therefore does not alter the local metabolic conditions, do not give rise to tumour formation. However, such an inert material as gold is, if arranged in the same manner as cellophane film, produces tumours. In experiments of KLEIN the tumours were induced by cellophane film in the A, DBA/2, C3H strains of mice and in (AxDBA/2)F$_1$ hybrids. No resistance was obtained in autochthonous mice, but syngeneic recipients showed weak immunity after preimmunization with irradiated cells. Irradiation of untreated mice prior to tumour inoculation reduced the size of the minimal inoculum in comparison with unirradiated recipients. This is a good indirect evidence of specific antigenicity of the tumour used. The lymph node cells from preimmunized animals showed neutralizing effects on tumour growth when previously mixed with tumour cells in vitro.

Relatively frequently, especially in mouse cells, spontaneous transformation occurs during cultivation in vitro. SANFORD et al. (1954, 1958) demonstrated the presence of a specific antigen in spontaneously transformed cells of C3H origin. Two cell lines, which were passaged in vitro and differed in their capacity of producing the tumours after application in vivo, possessed an identical TSTA. Cross-reactions were also observed with a tumour line which had arisen 10 years earlier. This suggests that random mutations in the antigenic configuration are not involved, but the oncogenic virus may play a role or participate in this process.

The antigenic specificity has also been demonstrated in tumours induced by using Millipore filters. The problem of antigenicity of tumours induced by hormones is still open. To the best of our knowledge, no such study has been published as yet in this respect.

Individual Specificity of the Tumour Antigen

From many aspects, the question of the extent to which the TSTA is common to the tumours of the same or even of a different aetiology is very important. This question has been conclusively solved for the tumours induced by the defined oncogenic viruses. A particular oncogenic virus consistently induces the same antigen, even in different species of animals. Different viruses are known to exist that induce cross-reacting antigens. However, it is difficult to decide whether or not related or identical viruses are involved which may differ only in the site of isolation. Most probably, even the so-called spontaneous tumours arising within inbred strains will possess a common antigen (KOLDOVSKÝ, 1961).

In tumours induced by chemical carcinogens, individual specificity has been detected by the majority of authors (cf. PREHN, 1965). PASTERNAK likewise observed individual specificity of tumours induced by physical factors (PASTERNAK et al., 1964). Nevertheless, cross-reactions were noted in isolated cases (PREHN MAIN 1957; STERN, 1960; KOLDOVSKÝ 1961). To explain these findings, SJÖGREN takes into account non-specific stimulation (1965) which can be so strong as to simulate specific immunity in some instances. Another possibility has been pointed out by PREHN (1965) — the tumours showing cross-reactions can really possess a common antigen which appears after superinfection with an endemically occurring virus. The possible presence of a polyoma antigen on methylcholanthrene-induced tumours has been suggested by SJÖGREN and HELLSTRÖM; the author was successful in obtaining cells with two TSTA's induced by two different oncogenic viruses (1967). Two tumour antigens may probably occur even after malignant conversion induced by a "naturally" arising hybrid virus SV40 and adenovirus (HUEBNER et al., 1964). The possible preimmunization with polyoma virus against a benzpyrene-induced tumour (SACHS, 1962) also suggests that this tumour has been superinfected with polyoma virus, or that a latent virus has been provoked by benzpyrene.

The individual specificity of TSTA of carcinogen-induced tumours is generally accepted, but it seems unlikely that as many TSTA's as carcinogen-induced tumours should exist. The number of such antigens seems to be definite and the individual specificity is given by the variability within the definite number of antigens. If e. g. 50 such antigens would exist, it may be possible, but with little probability, to find specifically cross-reacting tumours within a laboratory. This situation may be remotely similar to individual specificity of transplantation antigens within an outbred population. Here evidence of a definite number of antigens responsible for individual specificity has been provided by means of tolerance induction by a pool of cells from many donors towards any, randomly selected, individual of the same population (HAŠEK, HAŠKOVÁ, 1958). To determine the number of carcinogen-induced TSTA's, it might suffice to induce immunity by a pool of a certain number of tumours against any of the other tumours as has been suggested by PREHN (1965). Immunization of this sort might also specifically influence chemical carcinogenesis. The present state of knowledge makes it impossible to carry out such experiments with success. Above all, the quantitative representation of antigens in different tumours is not known; an antigen may be present in insufficient amounts, or conversely, a large amount of antigen may induce immunological paralysis. The development of immunological enhancement must also be taken into account. ADAMCOVÁ (unpublished) in our laboratory observed an increase in tumour growth rate after pre-immunization with a pool from as few as 9 tumours. The number of individual specific antigens in carcinogen-induced tumours does not seem to be too high. It seems unlikely that on application of a relatively large amount of carcinogen molecules the tumour would develop out of one transformed cell as a single cell clone. GLOBERSON and FELDMAN (1964) found that different clones of the same tumour were antigenically similar; the similarity was also observed by PREHN (1965) though not consistently. If antigenically distinct clones were present in the tumour, then the clone with poorest antigenicity, or the least represented clone to which no strong immunity was at first induced, should be selected much more frequently; thus an antigenic tumour would be rarely found.

Stability of Antigen

Normal transplantation antigens are very stable, genetically controlled characteristics of both tumour and normal cells. They are determined by dominant (or co-dominant) genes. The inbred strains of some animal species, especially of mice, are therefore capable of maintaining stability in their antigenic structure for a number of generations. Nevertheless, the antigenic make-up may undergo mutations leading to the occurrence of a new antigen or to its loss. BORGES and KVEDAR (1952) observed loss of antigen in the C57BL strain by following the alterations in transplantability of myeloid leukaemia Cl498 indigenous to this strain. This leukaemia has been 100% transplantable in the C57BL/6 (B/6) and C57BL/10 (B/10) strains, but some individuals from the B/10 breed showed natural resistance. From these animals, a new subline B/10-x was developed and subsequent tests performed in F_1 and F_2 generations showed that mutation of a single gene(antigen) might have been involved. However, with regard to later studies of LINDNER and KLEIN (1960), the number of antigenic(gene) differences detected by means of tumour transplantability, must be taken with some reservation. The latter authors found that two co-isogenic strains — A and ASW — differing in a single antigen controlled by the H-2 locus when tested with a tumour graft, displayed about 10 further weak antigenic differences when tested with skin grafts.

If mutation, leading to the development of a new, antigenically different line of animals, may occur, then it is well conceivable that antigenic alterations may take place in somatic cells, e. g. tumour cells. Mutation in transplantation antigens has been long detected. CLOUDMAN (1922) observed that two tumours from the same mouse have a different transplantability. A few years later, STRONG (1929) observed a similar difference in transplantability of two tumours which developed gradually in F_1 hybrids between two inbred strains of mice. He concluded that at least one of these tumours underwent mutation as a result of which the population of cells with altered antigenic (genetic) characteristics grew and thus the whole tumour was changed.

AXELRAD and KLEIN (1956) concentrated their efforts on a search for cell clones within a tumour which might differ in transplantation antigens controlled by the H-2 locus. They compared the transplantability of the primary tumours in F_1 hybrids and of their lung metastases in F_2 hybrids. In three cases, obvious differences were found which suggested that metastases developed from a cell clone other than that of the primary tumour. Whether or not heterogeneity of a cell population in the primary tumour does already exist during malignant conversion, or whether heterogeneity develops during the growth of the tumour cannot be decided by such experiments.

In view of the possible losses of TSTA, the loss of a normal transplantation antigen(s) should be briefly mentioned. Detection of the loss is difficult. It has been found that, for example, SaI tumour lost several blood group antigens controlled by the H-2 locus. Since the presence of transplantation antigens is determined by the same locus, this tumour might also have lost transplantation antigens.

Attempts have been made to make use of the antigenic mutation of tumours and of the possible increase in mutations by irradiation for detecting the genetic effects of irradiation on mammalian cells. In his first work on this point KLEIN et al. (1957) revealed mutation in the H-2 allele of the tumour of F_1 hybrids (loss of antigen) and an increased incidence of mutations after a dose of 400 r; further analysis showed that antigens need not be lost, but can be present in some masked form, and this facilitates a "false" tumour growth and simulates the occurrence of mutation.

Mention has been made of the possible loss of antigens of SaI tumour. It is the more interesting that TSTA could be demonstrated in this tumour even after several years of passaging.

Transplantability of the tumours does not change only by random mutations, but also by alterations which are generally called adaptation after temporary growth on an antigenically different host. If the tumour has a TSTA, then its growth in the so-called syngeneic host is virtually the growth in an antigenically disparate recipient. Such adaptations deserve brief consideration.

An "adapted" tumour can be obtained by passages in an antigenically disparate individual which is, for any reason, incapable of reacting against the transplanted tumour. This tumour can then grow in normal, fully reactive individuals. As a rule, the adaptation of the tumour is temporary and its strain specificity returns after passages in the strain of origin. Permanent adaptation was observed by E. MÖLLER

(1964) when the adaptation was performed for longer periods of time (more than 4 passages).

Barrett-Deringer reported that transplantability of tumour changed after passages in F_1 hybrids (1950) between a tumour-susceptible and a tumour-resistant strain. This phenomenon has been analysed in detail, and an extensive literature had accumulated bearing on its various aspects. The changes involved do not appear to be permanently genetically coded.

MOLOMUT (1958) described a reversible change in transplantability of SaI tumour passaged in incompatible mice by means of immunological enhancement. The SaI tumour could thus be passaged for 2 years in C3H, BALB/c and C57BL strains of mice, but the original strain specificity returned after several passages in mice of the original A strain. On the other hand, E. MÖLLER (1964) obtained permanent loss of strain specificity after four passages in F_1 hybrids and the newly developed non-specific tumour lines had a lower concentration of surface antigens controlled by the H-2 locus.

Likewise, passages in immunologically tolerant animals (MARTINEZ et al., 1960) lead to alterations in the adaptation of a particular tumour. The antigenic variability of lymphomas after passages in F_1 hybrids has been described in many papers by HELLSTRÖM (e. g. 1960). Changes in transplantability — strain specificity were also observed after passages of tumours on the chorioallantoic membrane of chicken embryos (MIRAND, HOFFMAN 1955).

In the light of these experiments on the fate of normal transplantation antigens that are relatively strong in comparison with TSTA, the stability of TSTA and the frequency of detection of the immune response seem to be remarkable. Mention has already been made of the stability of TSTA of SaI and of the tumours occurring spontaneously in vitro, as has been described in the experiments of SANFORD. Complete loss of TSTA is probably not very frequent, since if this were the case, then every tumour should become non-antigenic after several passages. The cells that have lost the antigen, would outgrow as a result of selection pressure even in the primary tumour, if the reactivitiy of the host has not changed.

Selection in non-preimmunized hosts may proceed slowly and its course may be hampered by the growing tumour which can reduce the host's reactivity specifically and non-specifically. We have therefore studied the fate of TSTA of a tumour passaged by means of a large inoculum in the recipients preimmunized against this tumour (KOLDOVSKÝ and SVOBODA 1962 a). The tumour was induced by benzpyrene and two passages were made in preimmunized hosts. Since the tumour retained its sensitivity to immunity as well as its immunizing capacity after the immune pressure applied, it was concluded that in this tumour the tumour antigen was relatively firmly fixed genetically. The tumour previously underwent several passages in normal animals and after passages in immune animals it showed better resistance to immunity than its original form. Since a certain dose of this immunoresistant variant induced the same state of immunity as did a several times higher dose of the original tumour, we believed that a paradoxical phenomenon occurred, that is, an increase in the amount of TSTA (KOLDOVSKÝ and SVOBODA 1962 b). However, later analyses of the relationship between the size of the immunizing dose and the degree of immunity revealed that with weak antigens the smaller dose of antigen was a better immunizing stimulus (KOLDOVSKÝ and BUBENÍK, 1964). A similar observation was made by Mc-

Khann (1958) with weak transplantation antigens controlled by the H-3 locus. The possible explantation of this paradoxical effect may be that the larger amount of antigen towards which tolerance relatively readily occurs, induces a state of non-reactivity in a major part of immunologically competent cells than the small amount of the same antigen. The resultant state of immunity is then determined by the number of cells that could have been activated, by the proportion of activated and "paralysed" cells. Hence the results of the initial experiments revealed a decrease in the amount of antigen in tumours growing against immunity which is in correlation with the finding that these tumours are more resistant to immunity. Similar changes were observed with TSTA of tumours induced by methylcholanthrene and also with another weak antigen — the so-called sex-antigen (Bubeník et al., 1966).

Globerson and Feldman (1964) studied the antigenicity of tumours induced by benzpyrene during their first passages. A decrease in antigenicity was relatively soon observed. The tumours from the third passage had already lost their immunizing capacity. Since they continued to be immunosensitive to immunity induced by the primary tumours, complete loss of antigen was not involved.

Thus, another question arises whether the tumour induced by carcinogens always contains a detectable amount of TSTA. This question has not as yet been answered unequivocally. The methods and the criterion used for the detection of TSTA are of decisive importance. At any rate, some tumours, especially some of the benzpyrene-induced tumours, appear to be non-antigenic whereas other tumours of the same aetiology are antigenic under the same experimental conditions. Old and Boyse (1962) observed that the number of non-antigenic tumours increased as the latent period between carcinogen application and the development of tumour was prolonged. In other words, the tumours growing longer against weak immunity of the primary host become better adapted, or a clone of the least antigenic, the least immunosensitive cells is selected.

The possibility of selecting various cell clones offers another explanation why TSTA of carcinogen-induced tumours need not be very stable. In these tumours, the TSTA is individual-specific for a particular tumor. By analogy to individual-specific tumours individual-specific clones of cells may exist within a tumour. The work of Globerson and Feldman (1964) and of Prehn (1965) have been referred to in the section on the individual sepcificity of TSTA. Prehn's experiments should be mentioned in greater detail here. In methylcholanthrene-induced tumours, Prehn found similar clones of cells and clones differing from one another. They were not precisely clones grown in vitro, but tumour lines obtained in vivo. Of these lines, 6 showed no differences in specificity, immunogenicity or immunosensitivity, compared to two original primary lines. Other lines were less sensitive or had an altered immunizing capacity. In two lines there was a difference in specificity, but the difference might have been due to the difference preexisting in the primary tumour. The author formulated the hypothesis "that the tumour which appears to lack antigenicity may represent a tumour in which the antigens are still present but secondary changes of an unkown kind have interfered with their capacity to immunize and/or have interfered with the cytotoxic effects of the immune reaction".

The stability of the antigen seems to be greater with virus-induced tumours. In a study of the stability of TSTA in polyoma tumours Sjögren (1964) compared 13 cell clones obtained in vivo from a tumour induced by polyoma virus as to their sensitivity to transplantation immunity against polyoma antigen. All clones had the same degree of sensitivity, although they differed in their karyotype and sensitivity to infection with polyoma or vaccinia virus. The same was true of the clone growing in vivo out of a minimal dose of cells which was 100 times that used for the other clones. Since the antigen was not too strong and immunoselection on non-preimmunized animals need not have been sufficient for the selection of a non-antigenic clone, SJÖGREN passaged two tumours against immune pressure. One of these was subjected to 42 passages and the other to 19 passage in mice preimmunized with polyoma virus. No change in antigenicity was observed in either case. On the other hand, one methylcholanthrene-induced tumour showing an exceptional sensitivity to polyoma TSTA, lost its sensitivity after 21 normal passages. In this case, the loss of properties superimposed on the phenotype of already established tumour cells was involved. The polyoma antigen thus appears to be a very stable characteristic whose loss, according to SJÖGREN, is not compatible with further viability of the tumour cell. In other antigenic systems, e. g. growth of heterozygous tumour cells against immunity directed against antigens controlled by the H-2 locus, the antigenicity decreases (G. KLEIN, 1959). However, the presence of at least one H-2 complex is necessary for the viability of the cell.

The stability of a polyoma-induced TSTA need not be so unequivocal under conditions other than those in SJÖGREN's experiments. At least three polyoma virus mutants are now known. The first two of them differ in their biological characteristics; one forms a large plaque in mouse embryo cells in vitro, produces high titres of haemagglutinins (HA) and is highly oncogenic for newborn mice and hamsters. The second forms small plaques, produces lower titres of HA, and is of lower oncogenic activity. No difference in viral antigenicity between the two mutants has been shown (HARE, 1964). The third mutant described by HARE and MORGAN (1963) was obtained from the small-plaque mutant SE-210-H⁺. This variant differs from the strain from which it was derived by the presence of a new antigenic determinant, by the inability to produce HA and a reduced oncogenic capacity. The two virus strains, SE-210-H⁻ and SE-210-H⁺, induce cross-reactive TSTA and have the same capacity to produce immunity against TSTA (HARE, 1964). However, the large plaque strain of DULBECCO fails to stimulate significant immunity against cells transformed by the above virus strains. It is of interest that the polyoma virus strain of Habel did not induce immunity against cells transformed with DULBECCO's large plaque virus (HABEL, 1965). If this large plaque strain is at all capable of inducing TSTA, its immunogenicity is not comparable to that of the antigen produced by a small plaque strain. Finally, the polyoma TSTA induced in hamster tumours does not appear to have the stability observed with mouse tumour antigens.

Some of the TSTA of Rous virus-induced tumors were shown to retain their antigenicity unchanged during a large series of passages (KOLDOVSKÝ, 1965). Sometimes, a decrease or adaptation in antigenicity is observed so that it is difficult to detect immunity to this antigen (HARRIS, 1967). It is of interest that the decrease takes place more frequently in rats which are considered to be immunologically more reactive than mice (HARRIS, personal communication).

In the light of the results described, the TSTA is a relatively stable, genetically fixed characteristic of each tumour cell; this holds for both carcinogen- and virus-induced tumours. In tumours induced by carcinogens, the TSTA probably occurs as the product of the altered genome of the cell under the influence of the carcinogen (the carcinogen is usually a mutagen too). This alteration is, to some extent, brought about by chance. Moreover, some balance between tumour antigenicity and host reactivity takes place during growth. This antigen, therefore, seems to be less stable than it is the case in many experiments. The TSTA of virus-induced tumours appears to be more stable. The viruses induce genetic changes leading to the formation of TSTA in a definite direction so that the alterations are antigenically specific for a particular virus. The alterations that did not arose by mutation, but by incorporation of the viral genome within the genome of the cell, or by virus-directed change of the cell genome, are less sensitive to external influences.

Considerations of the stability of TSTA, mostly detected by induction of transplantation resistance, have to take into account that resistance need not be detected, because the TSTA was lost, or the reactivity of the host changed. The first possibility has been discussed in this section, the latter will be paid attention in the sections on Tolerance to TSTA and Immunological Enhancement.

The Characteristics of TSTA

The TSTA is comparable in its biological properties (genetic control, ability to induce transplantation resistance, tolerance and formation of enhancing antibodies) with normal, better known transplantation antigens. Nevertheless, knowledge of normal transplantation antigens is limited as regards their subcellular localization and especially their biochemical properties.

The transplantation antigens have been revealed in almost all subcellular fractions by means of preimmunization. These fractions vary considerably as to their activity and immunizing capacity. A major part of the activity is localized in the cellular membrane, as has been shown in the experiments of GORER and MIKULSKA (1954) by the haemagglutination technique and in those of MÖLLER (1961) by the immuno-fluorescence technique. Localization of these antigens in the cellular membrane has also been confirmed by cytotoxic tests with allogeneic and heterologous sera. Studies of HOUGHTON (1965) indicated that a critical amount of transplantation antigenic activity (69—97%) was localized in the cellular membrane. The author made a quantitative comparison using the technique of absorption of cytotoxic activity, as has already been mentioned in the section on the Methods of detection of TSTA. Insofar as the activity has been detected by other authors in other fractions, this may be due to "contamination" of these fractions. For example, according to KANDUTSCH (1960), there are 3% of the intact cells in the nuclear fraction. In the mitochondrial fraction, aggregations of particles smaller than mitochondria may be present.

The views on the biochemical nature of the transplantation antigens are less uniform. This is probably due to the fact that the activity may be lost, the antigen may be destroyed during biochemical analysis. Lastly, the antigen may be a complex which is biochemically divided into two fractions. Perhaps each fraction may be suspected to contain transplantation antigens but recently the view has been taken that this may be an insoluble lipoprotein containing a small amount of carbo-hydrates (HOUGHTON, 1965).

While much remains to be learned concerning TSTA, its general characteristics seem to show a recognizable kinship with those of normal transplantation antigens. In experiments with benzpyrene-induced tumours conducted together with HILGERT (KOLDOVSKÝ, Dissertation Thesis 1960), the author pointed out that the lipoprotein fraction showed the highest immunizing activity. Further experiments extended to methylcholanthrene-induced tumours were carried out in co-operation with BUBENÍK and KRYŠTOFOVÁ (KOLDOVSKÝ et al., in press). The results on the activity of the lipoprotein fraction are given in Fig. 1.

Furthermore, the activity of separate subcellular fractions was studied in the model of methylcholanthrene-induced tumours (BUBENÍK et al., 1965). Transplantation resistance may be induced even if the antigens partially overlap, while almost complete antigenic similarity is necessary for the induction of tolerance. The afore mentioned studies on the activity of fractions were therefore completed with experiments on the induction of toler-

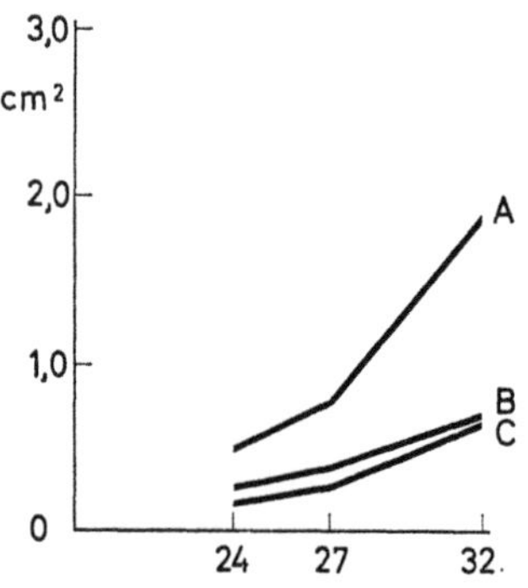

Fig. 1. Immunity to RVA 2 tumour induce with chicken Rous sarcoma and purified Rous virus. A—control; B—chicken Rous sarcoma; C—purified Rous virus

gradient were compared; the fourth fraction — the so-called soluble fraction was ance. Altogether three corpuscular fractions obtained by centrifugation in a sucrose the supernatant obtained by centrifugation at 105,000 g per 90 minutes. It can be seen from Fig. 2 that the immunizing capacityof the nuclear and microsomal fraction

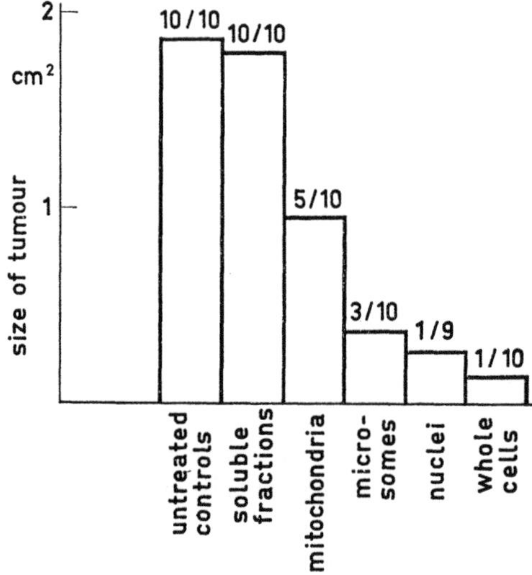

Fig. 2. Antigenicity of subcellular fractions of tumour cells

was similar to that of a whole tumour cell. The mitochondria were less effective and the soluble fraction practically ineffective. Experiments on tolerance induction also revealed the highest activity in the nuclear and microsomal fraction, whereas the mitochondrial fraction was not effective (Fig. 3, 4).

Mention has already been made that the presence of TSTA on the surface of cells is demonstrated by the cytotoxic test, especially in leukaemic cells. So far as a

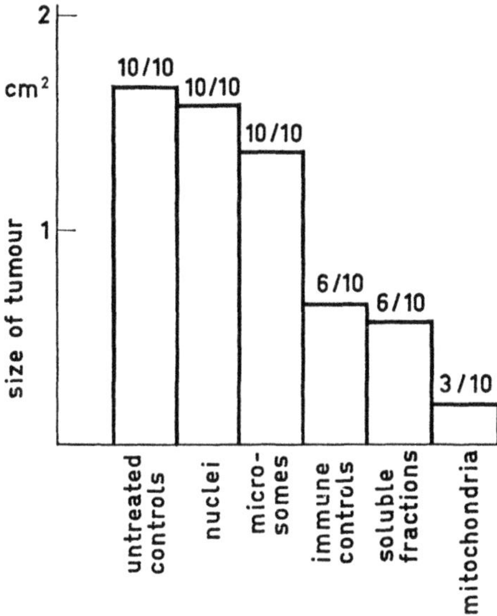

Fig. 3. Tolerance induced by fractions of tumour cells in adult life

tumour specific surface immunofluorescence (ring) reaction is demonstrated for some tumours, as has been observed by MÖLLER for the transplantation antigens controlled by the H-2 locus, one of the explanation is that the TSTA is responsible for this

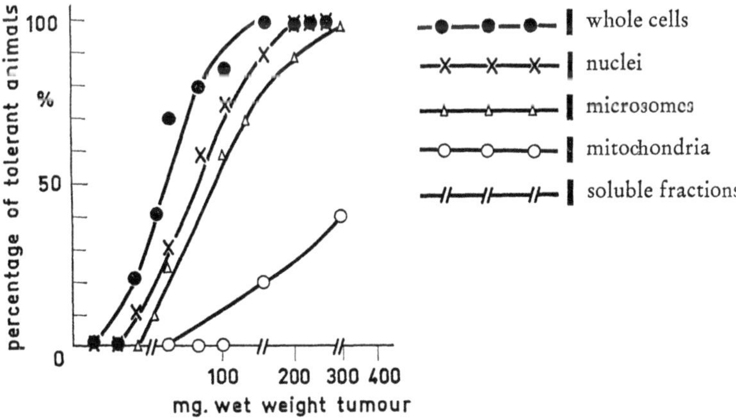

Fig. 4. Induction of tolerance to tumour antigen in newborn mice

reaction. However, if such tumours produce the virus, then the antiserum in which various types of antibody may be present, will detect the virus on the surface of cells.

Using heterologous rabbit antisera absorbed by normal tissues from mice of the same strain as the tumour, BRONDZ (1964) was successful in demonstrating a specific antigen in the cell membranes of two tumours induced by carcinogens — SaI (benzanthracene) and MCH2 (methylcholanthrene). The antigens were individually specific for each tumour. Antigens serologically detected in earlier experiments are frequently common to many tumours. Since the individual specificity of TSTA of carcinogen-induced tumours is a frequent phenomenon, it can be supposed that BRONDZ demonstrated the TSTA or its part by this method (BRONDZ, 1964).

MOLONEY (1965) demonstrated the TSTA in the microsomal fraction of Moloney leukaemia cells. DAVIES studied the X antigen in carcinogen-induced leukaemias and in some viral leukaemias and found it similar to transplantation antigens in its biochemical characteristics; the genetic locus determining the presence of TSTA also seems to be close to the H-2 locus. Finally, it has been found that the genetic control of TL antigen common to some leukaemias and present in the normal thymus of some strains of mice, is localized on the 9th chromosomal pair as the H-2 locus (DAVIES et al., 1966).

Little is known about chemical and physical influences that may damage TSTA which is probably as thermolabile (personal observation) as normal transplantation antigens; no relevant experiments, to the author's knowledge, have been reported. The tissue frozen at —20° C retains its specific antigenicity for several months (KOLDOVSKÝ, 1961). The tumours stored in a tissue bank at —79° C may retain their immunosensitivity. Carcinogen-induced tumours are known to possess TSTA resistant to doses of 14,000 R (REVESZ, 1960) and 20,000 R (KOLDOVSKÝ, 1961), whereas the antigen of tumours induced by polyoma and Rous sarcoma virus is more sensitive to X-irradiation. SJÖGREN (1962) found that immunity was very weak or could not be detected when polyoma tumour cells were irradiated with a dose of 8,000 R, while a live allogeneic tumour or the virus induced strong immunity against the same tumour. Similarly, the TSTA of RSV-induced tumours may be destroyed by doses above 10,000 R which produce no lesions to the TSTA of other tumours (BUBENÍK et al., 1966).

So far as the author is aware, the sensitivity of TSTA to enzymes or its stability with regard to chemical agents has not yet been studied.

The Relation of TSTA to Tumour-Specific Antigens Detected by other Methods

In opening this chapter, it should be pointed out that very little is known about this relationship. Comparative studies of various tumour antigens are rare and a number of earlier findings of tumour specific antigens based on serological methods require re-evaluation whether tumour specific antigens have really been involved. Recently, the data have been accumulated that antigens detected by agaroprecipitation as specific for the tumours, may also be found in normal tissues, be it embryonic tissue, the regenerating liver, or the digestive tract (cf. 2, ZILBER, ABELEV, 1962). Using the method of agaroprecipitation with heterologous rabbit antiserum ABELEV demonstrated a specific antigenic component in chemically induced hepatoma of the C3H mouse strain, and distinguished it from organ specific liver components persisting in the hepatoma. This specific antigenic component was obtained in very pure state by ABELEV's modification of the immunofiltration method. Its content in tumour tissues rose with the number of serial passages when the dedifferentiation and the degree of malignancy of the particular tumour increased. ABELEV tried to immunize the animals against the tumour with purified antigen but did not find any influence on growth of a syngeneic tumour, or the presence of cytotoxic antibodies against tumour cells in vitro. This is not surprising because the TSTA is probably not soluble and is therefore indetectable by agaroprecipitation. The hepatoma also contains specific antigenic components other than the mentioned agaroprecipitating antigen. The rabbit antiserum absorbed with normal and agaroprecipitating antigen consistently shows positive fluorescence reactions with hepatoma tissue (ABELEV and LEJNEVA, 1962). Further analysis revealed that the antigen involved was not a true tumour specific antigen but an antigen appearing in serum of normal animals after hepatectomy (during liver regeneration) or in embryonic tissues. [Taking into account the view expressed some time ago that rapidly growing tissues may have a certain antigen (enzyme?) in common (KOLDOVSKÝ, 1962), we attempted to explain some of our experiments on the individual specificity of the tumour antigen.] Although this antigen was found, for example, in embryonic tissues, it is possible that it may also be present in normal adult tissues and is indetectable with the methods available.

Two types of antigens have been demonstrated with certainty as antigens appearing only in tumours, both of them have been shown for tumours induced by oncogenic viruses. It is the viral antigen appearing in tumours producing the virus and the so-called complement-fixing antigen CFA. The latter must be distinguished from the antigen which is known to be detectable by complement fixation tests in tumour tissues of various origin since 1927 (cf. DAY, 1965).

It has relatively early been demonstrated that the viral antigen responsible for the formation of virus neutralizing antibodies cannot be identical with TSTA. Animals immunized, for example, with polyoma virus are resistant to subsequent inoculation of polyoma tumour, but this immunity is different from antiviral immunity (this question has been discussed in previous sections). The presence of virus neutralizing antibodies does not indicate the degree of resistance to tumours. For example, the animal cannot be resistant after immunization with inactivated virus (virus neutralizing or haemagglutination inhibiting antibodies may show high titres). Conversely, the animal immunized with an allogeneic, non-virus-producing tumour has no virus neutralizing antibodies and is resistant against a syngeneic tumour. Similarly, it has been shown for mouse tumours induced by Rous sarcoma virus that animals resistant against to tumour have no virus neutralizing antibodies, nor do the tumours passaged in immune animals have a decreased capacity to produce tumours after back-transfer to chickens (KOLDOVSKÝ et al., 1964). The latter experiment would mean that immunity does not influence the formation of the viral genome in mammalian cells.

Likewise, the CFA does not appear to be identical with TSTA, but seems to be identical with antigen detectable by indirect-fluorescence method in the nucleus of tumour cells (GILDEN et al., 1965). The TSTA has to be present on the surface of cells. This surface antigen can be demonstrated, for example, by means of a specific cytotoxic reaction with rabbit antisera in the presence of complement (TEVETHIA and RAPP, 1965). It is distinguishable from intranuclear CF antigen because hamster antisera reacting with CFA fail to react with surface antigens (RAPP et al., 1964).

Furthermore, no correlation between the presence of CF antibodies and resistance to the tumour has been demonstrated for Rous sarcoma (serving as an example of tumours induced by RNA viruses).

The question of the relationship between the specific antigen in leukaemias producing the mature, infectious virus and viral antigens is more difficult. An ingenious approach to this problem was made by PASTERNAK (in press) with Graffi leukaemia; he found that Landschütz sarcoma contained and produced the Graffi virus without any other alterations.

Mice resistant to Graffi leukaemia contain virus neutralizing antibodies and their serum gives positive fluorescence reactions with the surface of leukaemic cells. Similar positive reactions were detectable with cells of the Landschütz sarcoma. After antisera had been absorbed with Landschütz tumour cells, their neutralizing capacity disappeared, and the surface fluorescence reactions were negative with Landschütz cells, but positive with Graffi leukaemia cells. This experiment shows that two antigens are present on the surface of Graffi leukaemia cells. One of these is a cellular, virus-induced antigen probably identical with TSTA, and the other is viral antigen. The results with Landschütz tumour indicate that an oncogenic virus may be present in malignant cells, and is produced by them, but a new cellular antigen was not formed when cells of another origin were involved. This could suggest that the cellular antigen is not a direct product of the viral genome, but the outcome of the interaction between the viral and cellular genome.

Of pertinent interest is the relationship between CF antigen (CFA) and viral antigen. Virus neutralizing antibodies (and also the antigen) are different from CF antibodies. For SV40 it has been shown that CFA is a cellular component which is not associated with the viral particle or its subunits (GILDEN et al., 1965). This is the so-called early protein appearing a few hours before the viral antigen. On the other hand, CFA of Rous sarcoma (serving as an example of tumours induced by RNA viruses) may be identical with the internal viral capsid (PAYNE et al., 1966; KELLOFF, VOGT, 1966; BAUER, SCHÄFFER, 1965).

The specific antigenicity of tumours may also be demonstrated by means of the immunofluorescence test or cytotoxic reactions. Insofar as the fluorescence technique detects such antigens intracellularly (intranuclearly), the fluorescence antigen is identical with CFA. The surface fluorescence antigen (of the cell membrane) detectable on non-virus-producing cells is probably identical with TSTA. Likewise, the antigen detectable by cytotoxic reactions or adoptive transfer may be identical with TSTA.

The Mechanisms of Antitumour Immunity

It is of interest that the study of the mechanism of specific antitumour immunity has been developing along similar pathways as that of transplantation immunity. It has been shown for transplantation immunity both indirectly by morphological studies and directly by adoptive transfer of immunity by means of immune cells and by experiments with diffusion chambers that immune cells play a leading role in the destruction of allografts (cf. ALGIRE et al., 1957). Antiserum was supposed to play a minor role but recent experiments showed its importance in the rejection of grafts in the allogeneic system.

In the syngeneic system, the role of antiserum in the destruction of tumour grafts has also been denied, in spite of positive results obtained, in particular, in experiments using large amounts of antiserum. It is beyond dispute that immune cells (intracellular antibodies) play a decisive role in specific antitumour immunity.

The importance of immune cells has been confirmed by successful adoptive transfers of immunity against carcinogen-induced tumours (KLEIN, 1960; KOLDOVSKÝ, 1961) and by inefficacy of antiserum (KLEIN, 1960). The reaction of regional lymph nodes and spleen taking place during tumour growth (KOLDOVSKÝ, 1961; WOODRUFF and SYMES, 1962) also supports the role of immune cells in the host defence mechanisms against the tumour. The adoptive transfer of immunity has been successful with almost all tumours in which TSTA has been demonstrated.

Using a lymphoma induced by Gross virus, SLETTENMARK and KLEIN (1962) tested the minimal amount of immune cells capable of preventing tumour growth in adoptive transfer. They injected a certain amount of tumour cells to which various, but always several times higher amounts of immune cells from a control animal or an animal specifically preimmunized against a given tumour, were added. The proportion of 100—170 immune cells per tumour cell appeared to be most effective. However, it is difficult to say how many specifically preimmunized cells are really present in the suspension prepared from the spleen of the preimmunized animal. Their proportion is probably very small. The method of preimmunization is also important for the result of the experiment, because the more intensive the immunization, the greater the number of immune cells prepared. The above authors have really demonstrated that immune cells from long and repeatedly preimmunized animals gave better results than those from animals preimmunized only three times and shortly before collection of cells.

In experiments with benzpyrene- and methylcholanthrene-induced tumours OLD et al. (1962) found that the activity of various types of immune cells was different. On using the lymph node cells the adoptive transfer was successful even though immune cells and tumour cells were inoculated remotely from one another. Similar results were obtained in our laboratory (BUBENÍK, KOLDOVSKÝ, 1964). E. KLEIN and SJÖGREN (1960 b) obtained positive results only when tumours and immune cells were mixed in vitro prior to inoculation. In experiments on neutralization of tumour cells by immune cells from regional lymph nodes OLD et al. (1962) observed a similar situation as SLETTENMARK and KLEIN. If peritoneal cells from hyperimmunized animals were used, the proportion of 3 immune cells per tumour cell was sufficient to obtain positive results. Histochemical reactions showed that more than 50% of the cells used were macrophages.

In our experiments attention has been concentrated not only on the time interval between immunization and collection of immune cells or frequency of immunization, but also on the effect of the size of the dose. This question will be discussed in detail in the section on tolerance. In this place, only the experiment on adoptive transfer of immunity against methylcholanthrene-induced tumour in DBA/1 strain of mice will be described. Mice were immunized repeatedly with a large dose (300 mg irradiated tissue, wet weight) and yielded cells which were ineffective in adoptive transfer. Their non-reactivity was more apparent when compared with the effect of cells from donors immunized in the same manner but with much smaller doses (Fig. 5). Non-reactivity of cells from "paralyzed donors" lasted only 3 weeks.

Thereafter, there was a retardation in growth, and by the 30th day the tumours were twice smaller than those observed in control animals.

The break in the original curve is typical of the given experimental system, as has been confirmed in repeated experiments. These results were remarkable because retardation began at the time of tumour progression, the tumours reaching approximately 1 cm. in diameter. One explanation of this unexpected result may be that the cells used were immune and resistance was transferred. This was refuted by the observation that the tumours grew better in animals yielding the immune cells than in the controls, and that, after tumour and immune cells from resistant animals were mixed, a retardation in tumour growth was noted from the very beginning and not 24 days later. A second interpretation includes two possibilities: 1. Stimulation of the host reticuloendothelial system by transferred "non-reactive" immune cells. Such cells may transfer the tumour antigen or the enzymatic system necessary for antibody formation. This explanation has been suggested, for example, by MITCHISON

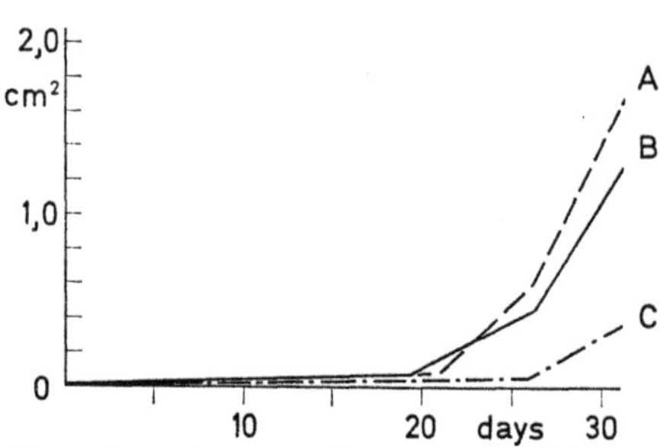

Fig. 5. Growth curves of tumour Mc2/DBA 1 after preimmunisation with large and small of this tumour. Curve A—mice immunized with 3×300 mg irradiated tumour suspension. Curve B—untreated controls. Curve C—mice immunized with 3×30 mg irriated tumour suspension. 10 males of DBA/1 per group

(1955) who obtained similar results in the allogeneic system. Another possible interpretation is that the mentioned time interval is the time necessary for immune cells, which are non-reactive because of being exposed to antigen excess, to recover when

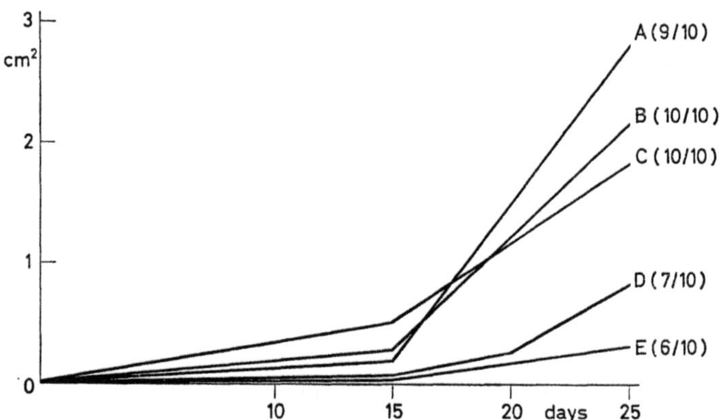

Fig. 6. Adoptive transfer of antitumour immunity with various immune cells when the donor mice have been immunized subcutaneously. A — controls; B — immune peritoneal macrophages 1:100; C — immune lymphocytes 1:4; D — immune lymphocytes 1:20; E — immune lymphocytes 1:100

they get into an environment without antigen. This explanation has been offered by OLD et al. (1962) for the results obtained with transfer of lymph node cells from animals bearing growing tumours.

A comparison of the results with transfer of immunity by means of lymph node cells (SLETTENMARK, KLEIN 1962) or peritoneal macrophages (OLD et al., 1962), insofar as the results obtained in different experiments are comparable, shows a greater capacity of peritoneal macrophages. This is somewhat surprising because small lymphocytes are generally considered to be the effector, the cell responsible for the destruction. The difference may also be due to the route of immunization. As has already been emphasized, not all immune cells from immunized animals are specifically sensitized. The ways in which immunologically competent cells come into contact with the respective antigen are important, too. Comparative studies were therefore carried out using the subcutaneous, suprascapular (close to the axillary nodes) and intraperitoneal route for immunization of animals. With subcutaneous immunization, lymph node cells were much more effective than peritoneal macrophages. The results of the experiment are presented in Fig. 6. Mice were given three immunizing injections of 50 mg irradiated MCl tumour suspension each. In adoptive transfer peritoneal macrophages were without any effect even if 100 macrophages per tumour cell were used. Regional lymph node cells given in a ratio of 20:1 showed a marked retarding effect, and in some instances were capable of preventing tumour growth. The effect was more pronounced with 100 lymph node cells per tumour cell. Using the intraperitoneal route, peritoneal macrophages were more effective than lymph node cells (Fig. 7).

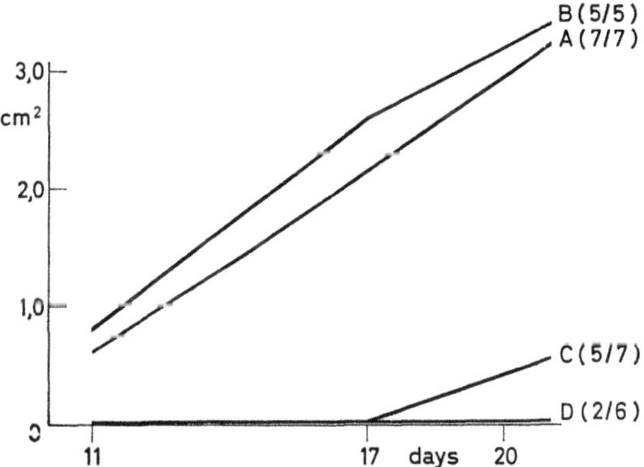

Fig. 7. Adoptive transfer of immunity with various immune cells when the donor mice have been immunized intraperitonealy. A — controls; B — immune lymphocytes; C — immune spleen cells; D — immune peritoneal macrophages

Although suspensions of immune cells washed by repeated centrifugation are used for adoptive transfer, the possibility remains that antibodies or antigen are transferred in the form which facilitates rapid immunization of the recipients. Negative experiments with cells killed by repeated freezing and thawing in a dry ice-aceton bath and in a warm water bath at 37° C indicate that the function of viable cells is really involved (KOLDOVSKÝ, 1961).

Theoretically, it can be assumed that cells may be sensitized in vitro against the tumour antigen. However, negative results with primary immunization in vitro against both weak and strong antigens excluded the possibility that immunization in vitro against a weak tumour antigen is easy. Lastly, it is known that tumour cells can be co-cultivated with heterologous immune cells. The conditions under which immunologically competent cells in vitro are really capable of performing their functions are not yet precisely known. Recently, a paper appeared suggesting the possibility of primary immunization in vitro under very exacting cultivation conditions.

In an attempt to develop a method for detecting the amount of TSTA in cell-free material, we tried to modify the technique of E. MÖLLER (1965) used for the

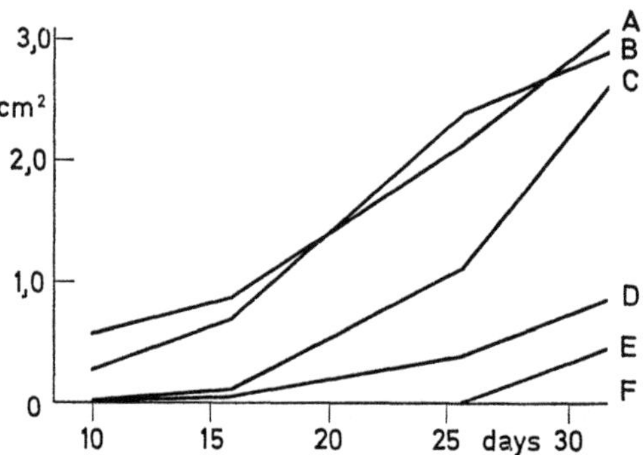

Fig. 8. Transfer of antitumour immunity by allogenic and syngenic lymphocytes sensitized in vitro against tumour RVA 2. A — control lymphocytes; B — allogenic lymphocytes on host preimmunized against these lymphocytes; C — allogenic lymphocytes mixed with tumour cells in ratio 40:1; D — syngenic lymphocytes mixed with tumour cells in ratio 40:1; F — syngenic lymphocytes immunized in vitro mixed with tumour cells in ratio 500:1

detection of the (relative) amount of antigen. MÖLLER compared the capacity of serum of known cytotoxic activity after absorbing it with material of different antigenic strength. The amount (relative) of antigen in a sample could be determined from the decrease in titre. Similarly, immune cells from one animal (or a pool from a group of animals preimmunized in the same manner) have a standard capacity for adoptive transfer. However, the attempt failed to remove the capacity for adoptive transfer using cell-free material containing the tumour antigen (KOLDOVSKÝ, 1967). In contrast, absorbed immune cells showed a greater capacity than non-absorbed immune cells. Absorption was performed with supernatant prepared from a tumour cell suspension crushed with sea sand. In the experiments, the tumours RVA2 and mice of the C57BL strain were used. As controls served immune, non-absorbed cells (positive controls) from immunized animals, immune, non-absorbed cells (negative controls) from normal animals and immune, absorbed cells from normal animals (control of the effect of absorption). It was surprising that not only absorbed cells from preimmunized animals were more effective in transferring specific transplantation antitumour immunity, but the same capacity was noted in absorbed cells from non-preimmunized animals. Experiments were repeated with lymph node cells, spleen cells and peritoneal macrophages. Identical results were consistently obtained. One of these experiments with lymph node cells will be described here. The cells sensitized (up to now called absorbed) in vitro showed a greater effect than cells from animals preimmunized in vivo. This can be seen from the course of the growth curves (Fig. 8) and from the number of "takes". Cells sensitized in vitro lose their capacity to transfer adoptive immunity when killed by repeated freezing and thawing (Fig. 9).

This speaks for the function of viable cells and against the possibility of antigen transfer (active immunization) by such cells. Despite this, a further control experiment was carried out, in which immunity was adoptively transferred by in vitro sensitized cells to newborn mice. These mice conceivably are not capable of reacting against the tumour antigen but ensure a good functional state of immune cells. In

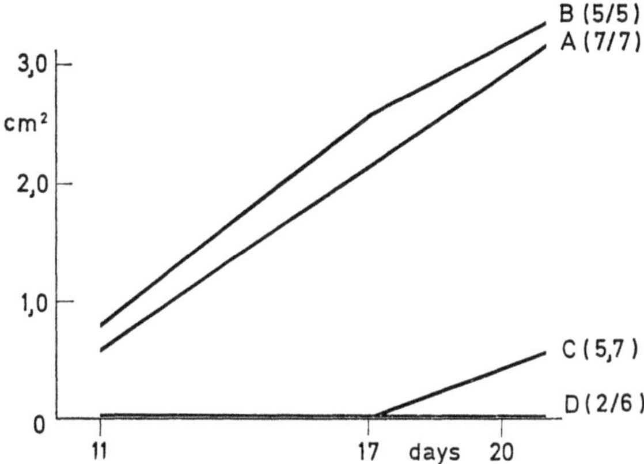

Fig. 9. Antitumour immunity transferred by lymphocytes sensitized in vivo and in vitro against tumour RVA 2. A — control lymphocytes; B — destroyed lymphocytes sensitized in vitro; C — lymphocytes sensitized in vivo; D — lymphocytes sensitized in vitro

this experiment, a marked retardation in tumour growth was again noted (Fig. 10). A further experiment confirmed again that the adoptive transfer is effected by viable functional cells. Allogencic immune cells sensitized in vitro which have a limited survival time in genetically foreign hosts, just as syngeneic cells, cause only temporary delay in tumour growth (Fig. 8).

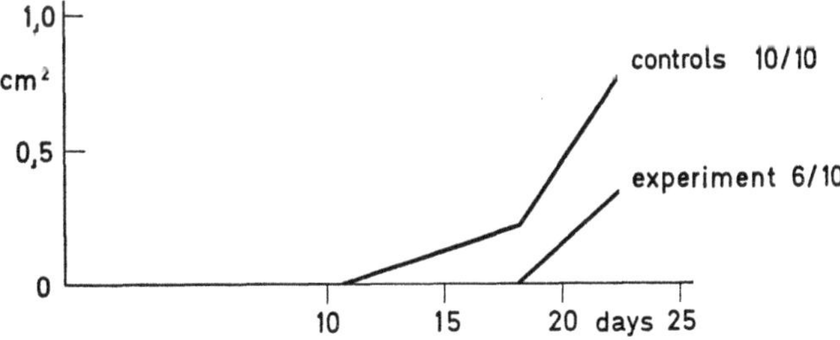

Fig. 10. Transfer of antitumour immunity by lymphocytes sensitized in vitro on newborna animals

Furthermore, the specificity of this reaction was studied and an attempt was made to demonstrate that the immune mechanism was really involved. We have shown that sensitization in vitro could be demonstrated against all the other tested tumours induced by both Rous sarcoma virus (as was the first tumour RVA2) and methylcholanthrene. The reaction was specific because the cells sensitized by one methylcholanthrene-induced tumour transferred immunity only against this particular tumour and not against any other methylcholanthrene-induced tumour that did not cross-react with the former (KOLDOVSKÝ, 1966).

HARRIS et al. (1956) showed that specific antiserum mixed with bacterial antigen (or cells) in vitro prior to the addition of immunologically competent cells (or antigen) prevented the interaction of antigen with cells, so that neither sensitization nor antibody production followed. We duplicated this experiment using the tumour RVA2 and antiserum from C57BL mice which were resistant to 50 minimal doses of RVA2 tumour. Antiserum mixed with cells simultaneously or prior to the addition of antigen prevented sensitization, but 30 minutes after antigen and cells were mixed, the antiserum was without any effect. Neither Serum from normal mice was effective (Fig. 11).

In adoptive transfer cells sensitized in vitro appeared to be more effective than cells from preimmunized animals. This was confirmed by the finding showing that lethally irradiated mice protected with cells sensitized in vitro (syngeneic bone marrow was also added) were at least as resistant against subsequent challenge with the corresponding tumour as mice preimmunized in vivo and not irradiated.

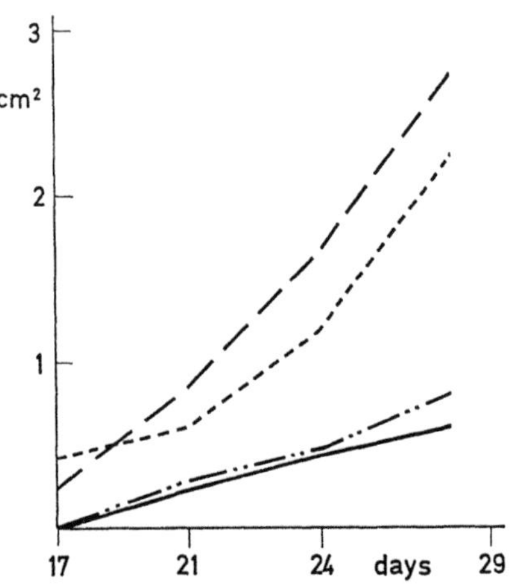

Fig. 11. Influence of specific antiserum on immune cells to be sensitized in vitro against tumour RVA 2. Curve 1—antiserum added to the cells before mixing with antigen; Curve 2—control serum added to the cells before mixing; Curve 3—antiserum added to the cells and antigen immediately after mixing; Curve 4—antiserum added to the cells and antigen 30 minutes after mixing. Ten minimal doses of tumour cells were used per mouse. Ratio of immune cells to tumour cells was 50:1. x: days after challenge. y: area of tumour in cm²

The most convincing evidence of immunological sensitization as a result of contact of antigen (TSTA) with immunologically competent cells would be the demonstration of a secondary type response effected by such cells. It has been demonstrated that animals protected after lethal irradiation with sensitized immune cells and bone marrow reacted to subsequent immunization with irradiated tumour cell suspension in the sense of an accelerated secondary response. Immunization was performed three weeks after the protection with sensitized cells. Control animals were protected with non-sensitized cells. Ten days after immunization all groups of mice were challenged with the respective tumour. Four groups were used: mice irriated with 850 R, protected with sensitized cells, immunized; mice irradiated with the same dose, but protected with control cells; only immunized mice, and untreated controls. The results are given in Tab. 1; where the growth curves correspond to individual groups of animals. In this experiment, as in other experiments with immunity against TSTA, it has been proved that immunity develops very slowly and is not detectable at 10 days after immunization. The mice protected with sensitized cells three weeks before immunization responded by secondary response.

The concept of the immune nature of sensitization in vitro has also been confirmed by other indirect proofs such as failure to sensitize cells from animals lethally irradiated 24 hours previously, or from animals specifically tolerant to a particular

TSTA. The in vitro non-reactivity in tolerant cells differed from that in vivo—tolerance in vivo could be longer detected than by using the in vitro method.

Recently, GINZBURG and SACHS (1965) demonstrated not only sensitization in vitro, but also the ultimate effect of rat lymph node cells on mouse tumour cells in vitro. The target cells were destroyed, the lymph node cells, which had already

Table 1. *Second set type of immunological response of cells from animals pretreated with in vitro sensitized immune cells*

Cells from mice	Ratio of immune cells to tumour cells		
	10 : 1	50 : 1	100 : 1
Irradiated with 850 r protected with cells sensitized in vitro, immunized, challenged	3/5	0/5	0/5
Irradiated with 850 r protected with untreated cells, immunized challenged	5/5	5/5	5/5
Nonirradiated, immunized challenged	5/5	5/5	3/5
Challenged	5/5	5/5	5/5

Ten minimal cell doses were used per mouse. The evidence was obtained from adoptive transfer.
Nominator — number of mice with tumour; denominator — total number of mice.

come into contact with mouse cells in vitro, gave secondary response. The reaction was entirely cellular in nature, the medium from cultures containing active cells had no detectable effect on mouse tumour cells.
The in vitro sensitization with subsequent detection of the function in vivo (by means of adoptive transfer) has the advantage that the metabolic background of the productive phase of immune response in vivo is ensured. The better effectiveness of cells sensitized in vitro compared to those from preimmunized donors may be explained by the fact that a higher percentage of cells can be sensitized in vitro than during immunization in vivo. It is, however, difficult to explain how sensitization in vitro takes place. (In general immunology, the question of which cells are sensitized and how, irrespective of whatever antigen is used is still open.) In adoptive transfer (also by means of non-sensitized cells) the in vitro sensitized cells come into contact with the tumour antigen, i. e., with intact tumour cells. As a rule, their effect on tumour growth is not manifest and the tumour grows at the same rate as out of an inoculum without admixture of immunologically competent cells. It is true that non-specifically stimulated immune cells mixed with tumour cells 500:1 are capable of retarding tumour growth (unpublished results), but it is difficult to say whether the retardation is due to only an extreme increase in the immune apparatus, or whether immunologically competent cells are, under these conditions, sensitized against tumour cells. Finally, it cannot be decided whether the growth of tumour inoculated in a mixture with a certain excess of immune cells is really normal. It is certain that the reactivity of immune cells against the tumour is markedly altered after 30 minutes' incubation with subcellular material from the same tumour. The explanation may be that the antigen in cell-free filtrate is present in a more "digestible" form; cells are sensitized at a more rapid rate than when immune cells have to take the tumour antigen from intact, tumour cells. The outcome is an accelerated reaction demonstrable by adoptive transfer.

The role of immune antiserum against TSTA in tumour growth is much less clear than the role of immune cells. While KLEIN and SJÖGREN (1960 b) and KLEIN et al. (1960) using immune cells transferred specific transplantation resistance against tumours induced by methylcholanthrene, attempts at passive transfer were negative. On the other hand, passive transfer with serum against benzpyrene- and dibenzanthracene-induced tumours was successful (KOLDOVSKÝ, 1961; OLD et al., 1962). In our experiments the following tumours were used: SaI (induced by dibenzanthracene), Bp3 (induced by benzpyrene in the A strain) and MC II (induced by methylcholanthrene in the CBA strain). Preimmunized mice served as donors of both immune serum and immune cells and thus the efficacy of both components could be compared. Serum in amounts of 0.3 ml/mouse was inoculated on day 0, 3 and 6 after tumour injection, immune cells in amounts equivalent to spleen cells and lymph node cells from one immunized mouse to one recipient mouse were given on the day and at the site the tumour was inoculated. With tumours SaI, Bp3 and MC II, antiserum significantly retarded the tumour growth, whereas immune cells prevented it completely in some mice. With spontaneous tumours of the CBA strain, antiserum was not effective and the transfer of immunity by cells delayed the growth. In the allogeneic systems, a paradoxical effect of antiserum is relatively frequently observed — that is, an acceleration in tumour growth. Immunological enhancement can readily be transferred by antiserum (the phenomenon of enhancement will be discussed below). Little is known of why in some cases enhancement occurs and in some cases resistance, why some serum transfers resistance, whereas another serum transfers enhancement and still another one is without any obvious effect. Of interest are the experiments of GORER and KALISS (1959) with three different tumours; under the same experimental conditions, enhancement was transferred by allogeneic immune serum against two tumours and in one tumour growth was retarded. In the syngeneic relationship, MÖLLER (1964) observed either retardation or acceleration of growth after passive transfer with antiserum against methylcholanthrene-induced tumours. The conditions determining transfer of resistance or enhancement by serum will be considered later.

Furthermore, the role of immune cells and antiserum has been studied in cells isolated from the host body, either in diffusion chambers according to ALGIRE, or in tissue cultures. The two components conceivably cannot be separated in the body, and if, for example, an inhibitory effect of antiserum is observed, it is difficult to say whether antiserum had a direct cytotoxic effect or whether an "opsonin-like" phenomenon was involved, i. e. antiserum only discriminated the tumour cells to be destroyed by immunologically competent host cells. In the early 1930's LUMSDEN (1931) studied the in vitro effect of antiserum on tumour growth. The heterologous antiserum was proved to have the greatest effect.

As early as 1933, Bisceglie made attempts to study the immune influence on isolated tumours growing in a colloidal sac. This technique could be fully developed when the filters of various porosity were produced which allowed the passage of essential metabolites into the tissues or cells examined but prevented the passage of host cells into the closed system. Thus the transplantats can be protected against an immune reaction and the tissue placed in a chamber does not elicit immunity. The technique was improved by using filters of cellulose nitrate of graded porosity whereby the mechanism of transplantation immunity could be studied in detail.

When the porosity was such as not to allow the host cells and target cells to meet, the transplant survived intact throughout the observation period (ALGIRE et al., 1957). Even the target cells were not damaged if placed in preimmunized hosts. When the porosity of the filter allowed the passage of host leucocytes and macrophages into the chamber with the target tissue, the target cells were destroyed. All types of cells that had penetrated into the chamber, did not participate in the destruction. Histological examination indicated that lymphocytes played a leading role. Destruction was not accompanied by phagocytosis. In further experiments, ALGIRE et al. (1957) inoculated immunologically competent cells together with target cells into one chamber. The target cells were destroyed only when cells from preimmunized donors were used.

The possibility of immunization with tissues placed in diffusion chambers depends on whether the antigen against which immunity is ascertained, is bound to cells and therefore fails to come in contact with the host. This is probably not the case with ascites tumours. APFFEL et al. (1966) showed that a considerable amount of antigenic material was localized in the ascites fluid of the Ehrlich carcinoma, EL 4 leukaemia, S-37 sarcoma and Krebs ascites tumour. BIGGS and EISELEIN (1965) found that the antigenicity of Ehrlich carcinoma ascites fluid resided within filterable particles. The antigen could be effectively removed by filtration through filters of 100 mμ porosity. The particles were proved to be a leukeumogenic virus even by biological tests.

There are experimental data supporting the hypothesis that immune cells damaging the target cells are also destroyed (CUDKOWICZ and COSGROVE, 1960). McKHANN observed a rapid transfer of H^3 thymidine from labelled immune lymph node cells into cells of ascites tumour against which the donor of immune cells had been immunized. This is regarded as indirect evidence of selective destruction of immune cells when they react against a homograft (McKHANN 1962). It can be supposed that the transfer of thymidine is accompanied by transfer of intracellular antibodies.

The role of small lymphocytes in transfer of transplantation immunity (and of immunity against TSTA) is confirmed by the possibility of transfering the graft-versus-host reaction (GOWANS, 1962). On the other hand, the formation of humoral antibodies could not be transferred by small lymphocytes, although a pool of spleen and lymph node cells was capable of doing so (VREDEVOE and HILDEMANN, 1963).

BENNET et al. (1963, 1964) and BENNET (1965) studied the conditions of phagocytosis of tumour cells in tissue culture. Peritoneal macrophages from mice phagocytized viable tumour cells in vitro in the presence of immune serum. Phagocytosis was also shown to take place when peritoneal macrophages were of the same origin as tumour cells, and antiserum was directed against antigens of both types of cells. Phagocytosis occurred even if antiserum was directed against the tumour cells, and the origin of tumour cells was not important in this case. Antiserum had both the opsonic and direct cytotoxic effect. The opsonic effect was also observed in diluted serum when cytotoxicity was no longer found. The phagocytized cells were viable as shown by vital staining using trypan blue. The phagocytized cells were, however, destroyed after a longer period of time.

Experimental results indicating that the target cells are destroyed by immune cells only when both these types of cells are in close contact, were supported by

HOLM et al. (1964). They found that this contact could be stimulated by PHA and thus the damaging effect was also potentiated. Similar results were obtained by E. MÖLLER (1965) with tumour and immune cells, and the contact of both these types of cells was increased by agglutination with inactivated rabbit antiserum.

The in vitro interaction of immune lymphocytes with tumour cells and normal cells was studied by BRONDZ (1964). He found that a specific immune reaction was involved. If cells from animals differing in strong H-2 antigens were used, the reaction took place even in the absence of complement and immune serum. The possibility of a specific reaction against an organ-specific (brain tissue) antigen of immune cells in vitro was pointed out by KOPROWSKI and FERNANDEZ (1962).

The interaction between immune and tumour cells was demonstrated by ROSENAU and MOON in 1961. From the point of view of specific antitumour immunity directed against TSTA, the recent work of ROSENAU and MORTON is of considerable interest (1966). They used tumours induced by methylcholanthrene in females of the C3H and C57BL strain and immune cells in the syngeneic relationship. Six tumours contained individual specific TSTA, two tumours occurring in the same mouse of the C57BL strain cross-reacted. The animals were immunized by intrasplenic injections and after 7 days cell suspensions were prepared from their spleens. Cell suspensions contained 90% of lymphocytes. In adoptive transfer of 200 immune cells per tumour cell, immune cells displayed the inhibitory effects on tumour growth. The same immune cells were added to 48-hour monolayer cultures of the corresponding tumour cells. The difference in the number of tumour cells was ascertained after they were mixed with immune, control (non-immune) cells and cells immune to another tumour. In one tumour in which the adoptive transfer was not effective, neither the in vitro experiment did show any effect on tumour growth. Growth of other tumours was inhibited by means of specifically preimmunized cells, whereas control cells and cells from animals preimmunized with a different tumour showed no effect. Microscopically, in addition to viable tumour cells, the remnants of tumour cells surrounded by lymphocytes were present by the 5th day after inoculation.

Recently, MATSUMOTO et al. (1966) studied immunity against spontaneously occurred leukaemia C-1498 of the C57BL strain. They found that resistance against this leukaemia could be induced in syngeneic mice by transfer of spleens from leukaemia bearing mice. Spleen cells from tumour bearers added to tissue culture were found on or around the tumour cells. The same behaviour was noted with spleen cells from resistant donors. Agglutination appeared about 3 hours after the addition of immune cells to tumour cells. The tumour cells contracted and condensed in feature resulting finally in cytolysis. The reaction was more intense during the next 18 hours, but some tumour cells remained intact. No agglutination was observed with spleen cells from normal mice.

Immunity and Carcinogenesis

In the preceding section evidence has been presented that experimental tumours contain the TSTA and that the organism is often capable of reacting against this antigen, and, under certain circumstances, of destroying the tumour. This antigen occurs at the same time as the cell is rendered malignant. Despite this, the tumour grows progressively until the death of the host. Spontaneous regression of really malignant tumours, in animals or in human beings, is extremely rare. It is difficult to estimate how frequent is the regression of a few malignant, transformed cells. Some clinical observations on the so-called dormant tumour cells suggest the existence of a regulatory mechanism which for years prevents the tumour from progressive growth. The malignant cells are known to be present in the circulation more frequently than it could be expected from the incidence of metastases. Spontaneous infection of mice with polyoma virus with subsequent presence of both antiviral (haemagglutination inhibiting and neutralizing antibodies) and transplantation resistance against polyoma tumour is direct evidence that cells were rendered malignant, but were destroyed before they began to grow progressively as an established tumour.

It seems of interest to discuss to what extent immunity may influence carcinogenesis. Specific immunization is successful only against tumours induced by oncogenic viruses. Here the situation appears to be more complicated because at certain age the animals are naturally resistant (probably on an immunological basis) against viral oncogenesis. In this direction, interesting experiments were carried out by DEICHMAN and KLUCHAREVA (1964) who found that resistance against SV_{40} tumour took some time to develop after inoculation of newborn hamsters with SV_{40} virus. Hamsters inoculated, as newborns, with SV_{40} virus and thereafter challenged with SV_{40} tumour cells are as susceptible (to these cells) as non-infected hamsters; challenge has to be done during the latent period of oncogenesis. After these animals are re-infected with the virus when immunologically mature, they acquire resistance to the tumour. The specific resistance develops even in the presence of a palpable primary tumour. This would mean that SV_{40} carcinogenesis takes place even though specific immunological tolerance is absent. Re-infection of animals with SV_{40} virus by the time the latent period terminates does not inhibit the induction of tumours in hamsters infected with the virus when newborn. However, the development of tumours is prevented when re-infection is performed in the middle of the latent period. This prevention is effected only by immunization with live virus and is specific.

Similarly, JONSSON (1966) showed that the reactivity was not reduced in mice bearing tumours induced by Rous sarcoma virus. This would mean that even in this case, the suppression of an immune reaction is not necessary for the development of tumour.

Mention has already been made of the role of tolerance to normal chicken antigens in RSV carcinogenesis in other avian species (ducks, turkeys) in the section on TSTA in RSV-induced tumours. Apart from Rous sarcoma virus, there exist the so-called RAV (Rous associated virus) and RIF (resistance inducing factor). These viruses are not endowed with the same transforming capacity as RSV, but are antigenically identical with RSV. It seems unlikely that they induce the TSTA although some of our preliminary experiments suggest it (unpublished). Tolerance induced by RAV virus towards RSV antigen in chickens (RUBIN et al., 1962) results in a greater and longer production of infectious RSV by the tumours developed. Whether this might influence carcinogenesis is not mentioned by RUBIN.

KLEIN and KLEIN (1965, 1966) found that carcinogenesis by Moloney leukaemia virus was influenced by specific suppression of immunity. Mice injected with homogenates of lymphomas induced by Moloney virus when newborn, showed a deficient or delayed antibody response, as measured by the indirect fluorescence test, in comparison with mice injected in adult life. In neonatally injected mice, there was a correlation between the appearance of antibodies and the length of the preleukaemic latent period. Control adult mice inoculated with Moloney leukaemia cells (allogeneic) form virus-neutralizing, cytotoxic antibodies and antibodies detectable by the fluorescence test (reaction of the cell membrane). The unresponsiveness of neonatally infected mice to immunization with the virus in the sense that they are not rendered resistant, corresponds to the concept of induced specific immunological tolerance to TSTA.

In our experiments, we did not attain RSV carcinogenesis in adult mice by specific suppression of immunity against TSTA of mouse Rous sarcoma (Annual report ICRF, 1966). Some mice tested for reactivity showed almost complete specific suppression of reactivity after the majority of animals in this experimental group were injected with material containing RSV. This finding confirms the observation of JONSSON that tolerance to RSV TSTA is not induced during RSV carcinogenesis. By this RSV differs, to some extent, from Moloney virus. Combination of specific suppression of immunity and cortisone treatment made it possible to produce carcinogenesis also in adult mice. Cortisone alone was ineffective.

Furthermore, experiments were carried out to influence immunologically carcinogenesis of spontaneous tumours. SHIUZO ISOJIMA and GRAHAM (1958) studied the effect of immunization on the development of mammary tumours in mice of the C3H strain. In the first experiment, with 22 mice, the spontaneous tumours were surgically removed and a small portion of them was left in the wound. The excised tumours were suspended in FREUND's adjuvant. Twenty-seven control mice were given FREUND's adjuvant alone. In experimental mice, the re-occurrence of tumour was significantly retarded. The authors believed that if a similar immunization were performed before the tumours started to develop, the incidence of tumours should decrease. This was confirmed in a further experiment, because at the age of 11 months 10% of the control mice and only 2.5% of the vaccinated animals had tumours.

On the other hand, HIRSCH and IVERSEN (1961) observed an accelerated development of spontaneous tumours after immunization. They used C3H and C3H backcross mice not containing the oncogenic agent. The latter mice were injected with the agent from C3H females when they were 27—36 days of age. Subcellular material from spontaneous tumours was used for immunization. In either case, tumour incidence was not reduced; on the contrary, the latent period of tumour development was shortened and the survival time of tumour-bearing animals was lowered.

Using the same strain of mice SCHWARTZ (1958) tried to prevent the induction of leukaemia by passive immunity. Antiserum was obtained by immunizing rabbits with non-cellular filtrates concentrated by centrifugation and incorporated in FREUND's adjuvant. This antiserum was administered to mice 24 hours before inoculation of viral material as well as on the day of inoculation and the next day. The tumour arose in 10% of the experimental mice and in 80% of control mice injected with serum from rabbits immunized with FREUND's adjuvant alone. This result can be accounted for by virus neutralization, and immunity need not have anything in common with immunity against TSTA. Furthermore, it was found that 50% of the mice injected with immune rabbit serum were resistant even against inoculation of live leukaemic cells.

Experiments on specific immunization against chemical carcinogens encounter the difficulties caused by individual specificity of TSTA of these tumours. There is a possibility of immunizing by a pool of several tumours, as has been suggested by PREHN (1965), who obtained but negative results; this method of immunization is associated with similar difficulties as polyantigenic preimmunization against carcinogen-induced tumours.

The fact that benzpyrene bound to proteins loses its effectiveness as carcinogen led Greech to perform experiments on immunization with complexes of isothiocyanate-benzpyrene and albumin. In his earlier experiments (1949) he obtained positive results, but later the influence on carcinogenesis was less pronounced (1952). In collaboration with ŠULA (KOLDOVSKÝ, 1960) we tried to duplicate these experiments and found that a conjugate of human protein with benzpyrene immunizes better than mouse proteins with benzpyrene. The results of Greech and the partly positive findings in our laboratory seem to be accounted for by experiments of OLD and CLARENCE (1959) on the effect of non-specific stimulation with BCG on chemical carcinogenesis. The immunological apparatus of the host is so increased by non-specific stimulation that he is capable of reacting against a few transformed cells and of preventing them, at least temporarily, from growing progressively. Thus, the latent period between carcinogen administration and tumour occurrence is prolonged in non-specifically stimulated animals as compared with the controls.

DECKERS used the microsomal fraction, which was shown to contain the tumour specific antigen (DECKERS et al., 1961), for immunization against cancerization. He found it possible to obtain a certain state of immunity against skin tumours induced by methylcholanthrene in rats immunized repeatedly with microsomes from the same kind of tumour (MAISIN, 1963). Upon replication of these experiments with dimethylaminoazobenzene (DAB), which produces hepatomas, he observed a higher incidence of hepatomes in some cases. The analysis of the conditions underlying retardation, or, conversely, acceleration of hepatoma occurrence after DAB showed that only washed microsomal fraction was capable of retarding cancerization with DAB. The supernatant of this fraction increased tumour formation as measured by the reduction of the latent period and also by the ultimate number of tumours. The microsomal fraction washed with 0.25 M sucrose was used.

Immunity can thus, to some extent, delay carcinogenesis. On the other hand, it is known (as will be discussed below) that the procedures reducing immunological reactivity may facilitate carcinogenesis. Some carcinogens (in the widest sense) appeared to be capable of reducing the immune response. The X-rays are generally known to have such capacity, but it is difficult to decide whether, precisely in this case, the suppression of immunity plays a major role.

VANDEPUTTE et al. (1963) found that polyoma virus injected into newborn (C3HxAKR) F_1 hybrids produced wasting disease. The degree of runting depends on both the dose of virus inoculated and the age of inoculated animals. The dependence on age may be associated with the possibility of virus replication and this indicates that the virus must attain a certain threshold level in the organs to induce runting. Histological examinations revealed the lesions in the lymphatic organs —

atrophy of PEYER's patches and depletion of lymphocytes in the lymph node and spleen cortex. Moreover, a decrease in the number of lymphocytes was observed in peripheral blood. These experiments indicate that the virus may be the primary cause of runting. These experiments may, but need not, mean that runting, which is practically an immune suppression of the host's reaction, may facilitate polyoma carcinogenesis. On the other hand, PARROT (1965) observed that spontaneous tumours appeared more frequently in mice in which wasting disease was induced by thymectomy and which survived long enough.

Survival of skin grafts in the combination of two mouse strains, which is usually 14 days, can be prolonged up to 2 months by application of methylcholanthrene (LINDNER, 1962). Secondary death resulting from irradiation can also be prevented by injecting lethally irradiated recipients simultaneously with allogeneic bone marrow cells and methylcholanthrene (RUBIN, 1960). The same effect of methylcholanthrene on survival of skin grafts was observed by LINDNER (1961). The work of DAVIDOVSKA et al. (1956) shows that the immune response need not always be suppressed — methylcholanthrene reduces the immune response against human erythrocytes in the DBA/2 strain of mice but not in the DBA/1 strain. MALMGREN et al. (1952) compared the effects of various carcinogens on the formation of haemolysins against sheep erythrocytes in mice. All the carcinogens studied, such as methylcholanthrene, benzanthracene, benzanthrene, chlorethylcarbonate, reduce this response and non-carcinogenic analogues are ineffective. On the other hand, if a relatively well reacting animal — the rabbit, and human serum albumin as antigen, were used, antibody formation could not be inhibited by methylcholanthrene (WILSON et al., 1966). BALL et al. (1966) found that the injection of 60 mg dimethylbenzanthracene into newborn mice resulted in a high percentage of thymomas. The incidence depended on the dose of tumour cells. With 60 mg the incidence of tumours was 90%; when the dose was reduced, the incidence decreased up to 19% for 10 mg. At the same time it was found that the administration of this carcinogen suppressed the formation of antibody against antigen given 4—11 weeks after application of carcinogen.

The effect of methylcholanthrene on immune responses in mice was studied in detail by STJERNSWÄRD (1966). He assayed the antibody cellular response by the technique of JERNE. This technique makes it possible to estimate the production of antibody by a single immune cell because this cell derived from an animal preimmunized against sheep erythrocytes produces lysis of sheep erythrocytes in agar. This lysis is manifested by plaque formation and the activity of spleen cells may be expressed as the number of plaque forming spleen cells (PFC). As early as two days after injection of methylcholanthrene, immunization with erythrocytes produced only a 50% activity of PFC of spleen cells as compared with the controls. After a single injection of methylcholanthrene the PFC remained suppressed during the whole latent period of tumour development. The decrease of immune response towards the graft differing in one antigen controlled by the H-1 locus (weak transplantation antigen) could not be demonstrated until the tumours appeared. The survival of skin grafts was not influenced in the preceding periods (STJERNSWÄRD, 1965). In a further work, using the same technique STJERNSWÄRD compared the effect of carcinogenic and non-carcenogenic carbohydrates on the occurrence of antibody forming cells. He studied the effect of benzo(a)pyrene, dimethylanthracene and methylcholanthrene as carcinogenic agents and anthracene and benzo(e)pyrene as non-carcinogenic analogues on the formation of immune cells on day 5, 11 and 36 after the administration of these carbohydrates. All the carcinogens showed immunodepressive effects. No such effects were observed with non-carcinogenic carbohydrates; this suggests that a correlation exists between the carcinogenic strength and the inhibition of the host immune response. The immunodepressive effects may favour the occurrence of antigenic tumour cells (STJERNSWÄRD, 1966).

The role of immunosuppression in chemical carcinogenesis after the administration of methylcholanthrene was studied by PREHN (1963). He demonstrated that methylcholanthrene given in the dose necessary for the induction of tumours could depress a weak immune reaction of the transplantation type against sex-linked antigen. The same carcinogen was proved to facilitate the growth of the first tumour passage in syngeneic mice. The transplantability of primary tumours is known to depend on their antigenicity. Another way of reducing the reactivity of the recipients of such tumours — e. g. whole-body irradiation — also facilitates their growth. In further experiments PREHN studied the direct effect of methylcholanthrene on carcinogenesis. A secondary injection of methylcholanthrene accelerated the development of tumours after the injection of the primary methylcholanthrene pellet localized at a distant site.

A number of works were concerned with the effect of thymectomy on the induction of tumours. MARTINEZ (1964) studied the effect of thymectomy performed at the age of 6 days on the occurrence of spontaneous mammary carcinomas in the C3H strain of mice. It is of interest that in thymectomized animals the percentage of tumours was significantly reduced and the time of tumour appearance was prolonged. This might have been caused by disturbed hormonal stimulation that is normally necessary for a spontaneous occurrence of such tumours. Otherwise this result is difficult to explain. Nevertheless, it should be borne in mind that in this tumour-host relationship the immune response against the tumour may be completely suppressed by natural tolerance (see section on "Tolerance"). The effect of thymectomy on the appearance of tumours of the lymphatic apparatus (thymectomy being also capable of preventing the occurrence of tumours — cf. MILLER et al., 1963) is beyond the scope of this review and will not be discussed here.

Immunological depression resulting from thymectomy may be restored by inoculation of intact thymuses. As shown by MAISIN (1964), the inoculation of intact thymuses combined with methylcholanthrene administration decreased tumour incidence in experimental animals as compared with the controls. One of the possible explanations is that reduced reactivity after methylcholanthrene was restored by thymus transplantation.

Mice of the C57BL strain are known to be more resistant to polyoma virus carcinogenesis than other mouse strains (DAWE et al., 1959). This resistance seems to be controlled genetically. The tumour incidence in F_1 and F_2 hybrids and the backcross progeny of a tumour-susceptible and a tumour-resistant strain of mice (JAKKOLA, 1965) support the assumption that the tumour resistance of the C57BL strain is an incompletely dominant characteristic of relatively simple inheritance controlled by not more than 2—3 independent genes. Similar results were obtained by CHANG and HILDEMAN (1964). This resistance depends on the whole body. The in vitro cultivated cells derived from all strains are equally sensitive to virus transformation. Experiments with thymectomy suggest that this resistance is influenced by the immunological reactivity of the host's organism. MALMGREN et al. (1964) found that neonatally thymectomized C57BL mice were equally sensitive to polyoma virus oncogenesis as the other strains. Similarly, the C3H mice susceptible to S strain of polyoma virus, but relatively resistant to the M strain, were fully susceptible to the M strain following thymectomy.

The reduction of reactivitiy by another treatment also allows the polyoma virus to produce tumours in C57BL mice. Inoculation of tissue extracts from the lungs of sheep suffering from pulmonary adenomatosis causes destruction of lymphoid tissues. Injections of these extracts together with polyoma virus increase the damaging effect on lympho-reticular tissues and produce tumours in a high percentage of animals with a relatively short latent period. This treatment also considerably prolongs the period of immunological unresponsiveness (TER-GRIGOROV and IRLIN, 1964). Adenovirus 12 has a low oncogenic activity and fails to induce tumours in some strains (YABE et al., 1964). However, if its application is combined with neonatal thymectomy of mice, then the tumours appear in a certain percentage of mice, while the controls remain without tumours (KIRSCHSTEIN, 1964). DEFENDI and ROOSA (1964, 1965) studied the effect of thymectomy on viral (polyoma) and chemical carcinogenesis (methylcholanthrene, dibenzanthracene) and also found an increased incidence of tumours after thymectomy. The thymectomized animals were less resistant to tumour grafts.

The Syrian hamster males are more resistant to Adenovirus 12 oncogenesis than females. Susceptibility of males can be increased by thymectomy (YOHN, 1965).

VANDEPUTTE and DE SOMMER (1962) found that the rats thymectomized neonatally and inoculated with polyoma virus at different ages were much more susceptible to viral oncogenesis than control rats. Since neither more virus nor a higher titre of HI antibodies can be demonstrated in the tissues of thymectomized animals, an increased incidence of tumours may be due to reduced reactivity against TSTA rather than to a higher virus replication. Similar results with chemical carcinogenesis were obtained, for example, by GRANT and MILLER (1965), and with polyoma carcinogenesis by RYOICHI MORI et al. (1966). L. LAW (1966) found that thymectomy performed at the age of 3 days had a great effect on the appearance of tumours, although the immune deficiency of such animals is subtle and not readily detectable by the common methods.

As a rule, the induction of tumours in mammals by means of Rous sarcoma virus is successful only when the virus-producing material (chicken tumour tissue) is inoculated into newborn animals. If this material is injected into adult animals, no tumours arise. KLEMENT (1965) was successful in inducing tumours in adult rats only when some milliliters of a fresh 50% chicken sarcoma suspension were inoculated. This dose could cause either specific immunological paralysis or non-specific exhaustion of the host immune reactivity which by itself might facilitate carcinogenesis in the given experiment. Moreover, specific immunological non-reactivity may be more readily induced in a non-specifically exhausted host (LAICOPOULUS and GOOD, 1964). Combination of thymectomy with irradiation makes it possible to induce tumours with Rous sarcoma virus even in adult mice (KOLDOVSKÝ and SVOBODA, 1965). Mice of the C57BL strain were thymectomized at the age of 6 weeks; 8 days later, they were irradiated with a whole-body dose of 350 r. A few hours after irradiation, they were inoculated with a freshly prepared suspension of chicken sarcomas induced either by the SCHMIDT-RUPPIN or the Prague strain of Rous virus. As control groups served: 1. mice inoculated with chicken sarcomas, 2. mice injected with these tumours after irradiation, 3. mice after thymectomy. On using the SCHMIDT-RUPPIN strain the tumours arose in 8 out of 28 thymectomized and irradiated mice, and only in 1 out of 17 irradiated mice. No tumours developed in the other groups when the Prague strain was used. Two tumours induced in the experimental group were further analysed and were shown to contain the RSV genome and the TSTA specific for mammalian RSV-induced tumours.

The fact that the tumours induced by methylcholanthrene possess the TSTA and that thymectomy reduces immunological reactivity and facilitates methyl-cholanthrene carcinogenesis has led BALNER and DERSTJANT (1966) to carry out experiments on whether the tumours induced in thymectomized mice are more antigenic than those induced in the controls. Prior to the application of carcinogen, they assessed the immunological reactivity of each mouse by means of allogeneic skin grafts. Thymectomized mice with normal reactivity were thus distinguishable from those with reduced reactivity. Although the numbers of animals in the thymectomized group with reduced reactivity and methylcholanthrene treatment were not large because of many deaths of experimental animals, it could be concluded that they displayed the same susceptibility to carcinogenesis as control animals. The antigenicity of tumours obtained was estimated using a relatively insensitive method, i. e., temporary growth of tumour, which was later surgically removed (FOLEY, 1953). Even with this method, they found significant differences between tumours developing in the experimental and control group. In the experimental group, 9 out of 10 tumours were highly antigenic, whereas a similar antigenicity could be proved in only 5 of the 10 control tumours.

Similar experiments were carried out by the author and Dr. PARROT (in preparation), but methylcholanthrene or Rous sarcoma virus were injected shortly after thymectomy. Antigenicity was compared in tumours after the first passage (the tumours were stored in a tissue bank). In methylcholanthrene-induced tumours the antigenicity was compared by the capacity of various doses of non-repopulating tumour material for preimmunization, in RSV-induced tumours (containing a common TSTA) by their capacity to overcome immunity induced in the same way. With methylcholanthrene-induced tumours, no difference was found between experimental and control group as to their incidence or antigenicity. The difference was significant for tumour incidence after administration of RSV; in no case was the tumour obtained in the control group because mice aged several days were injected. However, the antigenicity of tumours in thymectomized animals did not differ from that of primary tumours obtained in other experiments.

Tolerance to TSTA

On the basis of the experience obtained in many experiments on induction of immunological tolerance to biochemically defined and tissue antigens the following conditions may be defined: The ease with which tolerance can be induced depends on the age of the recipient — the younger the recipient, the easier the induction of tolerance. Tolerance to "weak" tissue antigens is more readily induced; that is, tolerance is difficult to induce in the combination of two mouse strains differing in many strong transplantation antigens, but relatively easy among individuals differing in weak transplantation antigens (controlled by the H-3 locus, sex-linked antigens). The phylogenetic distance may also be important — the more distant the antigen from the recipient, the more difficult the induction of tolerance. Tolerance may disappear with time. Using larger, and especially repeated doses, tolerance is more readily obtained and persists longer. The use of sufficiently large doses makes it possible to induce tolerance to some antigens even in adult life. Doses of antigen capable of maintaining tolerance are relatively small and do not differ from those which elicit a state of immunity in untreated individuals (cf. HAŠEK et al., 1961).

The TSTA is a very weak transplantation antigen, closely related phylogenetically; when the tumour grows progressively, the host organism may be regularly overwhelmed with an excess of this antigen. It can therefore be assumed that tolerance to TSTA may comparatively readily be induced and the growth of tumour is facilitated. Experiments were started to study the induction of tolerance to TSTA of benzpyrene-induced tumours in the A strain (KOLDOVSKÝ and SVOBODA, 1962). The tumour designated Bp7/A was produced in a male mouse and was in its 8th passage at the time the experiments started. Resistance was elicited using cell suspensions irradiated with 20,000 r. Animals were immunized twice with a dose of 40 mg per mouse. Since the repopulation of all tumour cells was not prevented by irradiation and the tumour injected into newborn animals began to grow in some instances, the irradiation was combined with freezing and thawing (three times) the tumour cells in a bath of acetone and solid CO_2 and in a water bath at 37° C. Sometimes the irradiated suspension appeared to be toxic for newborn mice, but its toxicity was removed by washing the suspensions repeatedly with saline. Experiments on tolerance induction were carried out in two groups of newborn mice — the first was injected daily with 20 mg wet weight non-proliferating material of tumour Bp7/A for the first three days of life, and the other with 20 mg suspension administered once only. 24 mice in the first group and 21 mice in the second group reached the age of 10 weeks. The third group consisted of control mice immunized in the same way as the first two groups at 10 and 13 weeks of age with 40 mg of irradiated suspension. The last group were untreated mice. The challenge dose grew progressively and led to the death of all tolerant and untreated animals. Only immunized mice were resistant (17 out of 20). Tolerance was also reflected in the rate of tumour growth. Tolerant animals died much more rapidly (48 ± 1.9 days or 52.0 ± 2.6 days) than untreated animals (64.8 ± 2.8 days). Interesting results were obtained in an experiment on the effect on adult animals of a large immunizing dose compared with a several times smaller dose usually used for immunization. While the small dose produced resistance to the tumour in 90% of the animals, all animals immunized with the large dose died. The growth curves showed that the tumour grew more rapidly in this group than in untreated controls (Tab. 2). For one thing, experiments on tolerance induction in newborn mice revealed that the antigen used for immunization after treatment, such as irradiation and freezing and thawing, remains fully antigenic and can induce tolerance. Tolerance to TSTA is relatively easy to induce and is long-lasting. The large dose of antigen given in adult life that resulted in an accelerated growth of subsequent inoculum, might have caused either immunological paralysis or immunological enhancement.

Table 2. *Influence of large dose of tumor antigen applicated to adult mice on growth of tumor Bp [7]/A*

Immunisation	Challenge dose	Total number of animals number of takes	%
2×40 mg [a]	0,2 ml 1% [b]	$\frac{10}{1}$	10
2×100 mg	0,2 ml 1%	$\frac{10}{10}$	100
Controls	0,2 ml 1%	$\frac{38}{40}$	95

[a] Wet weight of the tumor. [b] Untreated tumor cell suspension.

Attempts of neutralization by antisera from mice resistant against tumour RVA 2 of C57BL strain mice

Dilution of chicken RSV sarcoma extract	Days after inoculation 10 immune	control	15 immune	control	20 immune	control
10^{-5}	0/3	0/3	1/3	3/3	2/3	3/3
10^{-4}	0/4	0/2	3/4	2/2	4/4	2/2
10^{-3}	0/4	1/4	3/4	4/4	4/4	4/4
10^{-2}	0/4	0/3	3/4	3/3	4/4	3/3
10^{-1}	1/4	1/4	4/4	4/4	4/4	4/4

Nominator — number of mice with tumour; denominator — total number of chicken.

Adoptive and passive transfer from mice injected with tumour material

Dose administered to newborn mice in mg	Transfers Serum treated	untreated	Lymph node cells treated	untreated
20	7/11	7/7	1/14	14/14
100	10/10	14/14	10/10	14/14

Adoptive and passive transfers from adult mice treated by large doses of tumour antigen

Group	Transfers Serum treated	untreated	Lymph node cells treated	untreated
nuclei	6/6	6/6	7/7	5/5
microsom.	6/6	5/5	7/7	5/5
mitoch.	4/6 [a]	4/4 [a]	0/7	5/5
soluble fraction	6/6 [a]	6/6 [a]	1/7	6/6
immune controls	—	5/5	—	1/7

[a] Significant difference in growth curves between experimental and control mice.

Further experiments were therefore designed to study the conditions underlying induction of tolerance (immunological paralysis), enhancement or resistance. Experiments on enhancement will be described in the next section. In methylcholanthrene-induced tumours (BUBENÍK and KOLDOVSKÝ, 1964), the dose ten times greater than the optimal immunizing dose causes an accelerated growth of a subsequent inoculum. The difference between the immunizing and paralysing dose is greater than that observed in benzpyrene-induced tumours (Bp7/A); this is conceivable because the TSTA of methylcholanthrene-induced tumours is usually stronger than TSTA of benzpyrene-induced tumours. The relationship between the size of the dose used for immunization and the percentage of resistant animals was investigated in detail. Groups of mice of the C57BL strain consisting of 5—10 animals each were immunized with heavily irradiated suspensions of methylcholanthrene-induced tumour MC 1. Mice were given a single dose ranging between 5 and 600 mg. Eight weeks after immunization all animals

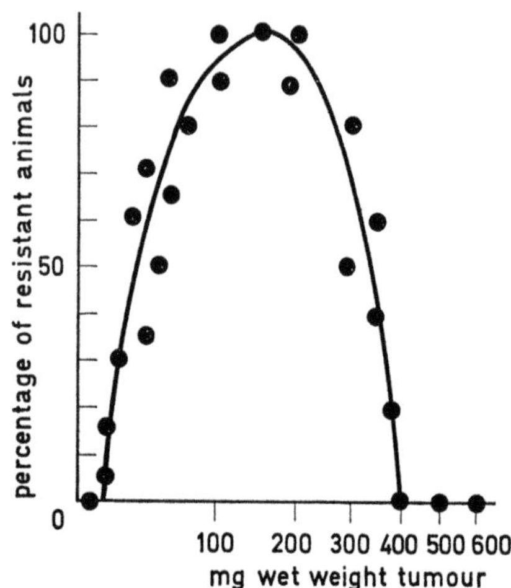

Fig. 12. Dependence of resistance on pre-immunizing dose of antigen

were challenged. The percentage of resistant animals rose as the dose increased (Fig. 12); almost a 100⁰/o resistance was obtained when the dose of 100 to 200 mg per mouse was used in this experimental system. On increasing further the immunizing dose, the per-

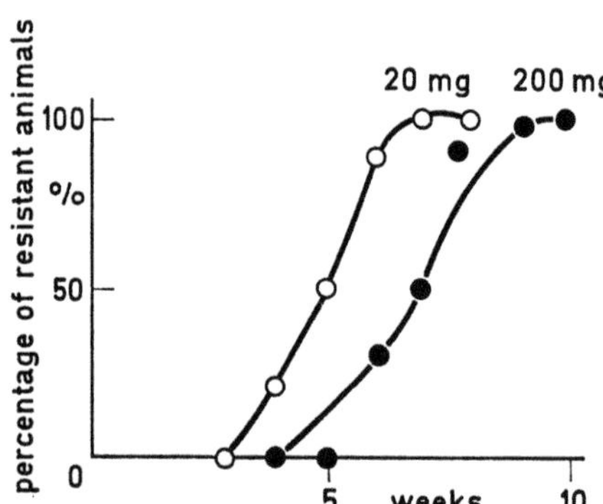

Fig. 13. Dependence of resistance on dose and time interval

centage of resistant animals fell — the doses of 500 mg and more did not induce any resistance, but stimulated the tumour growth. Analogous results were obtained with two different tumours induced by methylcholanthrene in another two strains.

Furthermore, attention was paid to the relationship between resistance and the time interval between immunization and challenge. The tumour MC 1 and groups of 5 to 10 mice preimmunized with a single dose of 20 or 200 mg heavily irradiated cell suspension were again used. After immunization mice were tested at weekly intervals. As can be seen from Fig. 13, the percentage of resistant animals increased as the time interval between immunization and challenge was prolonged. With the dose applied, it was apparent that the greater the immunizing dose, the longer the interval required for the induction of resistance.

The same tumour — MC 1, which was found to be strongly antigenic from the point of view of TSTA, was used for the induction of tolerance in newborn mice. Both various doses of irradiated cells and their subcellular fractions were used. At the age of 6—7 weeks tolerant mice and untreated controls were immunized with a single dose of 50 mg irradiated suspension. After another 7—10 weeks, both these groups and a further group of untreated mice were challenged. Some mice were not challenged, but their serum and lymph node cells were collected on the day of challenge and their capacity for passive and adoptive transfer was investigated. A single dose of 100 mg irradiated suspension given within 24 hours of birth resulted in tolerance in 90% of the animals. Tolerance proved to be specific because mice tolerant to tumour MC 1 reacted against another tumour of the same strain (Bp 1 induced by benzpyrene) as control mice did. Both serum and immune cells from tolerant animals showed no effect on tumour growth in untreated animals.

Using the same doses as in experiments with Bp7, attempts to induce immunological paralysis in adult mice (tolerance to tumour MC 1 in adult life) failed. The inoculation of as much as gramme quantities (in 4—5 injections) resulted in tumour growth. Tolerance was induced by repeated injections of subcellular fractions. Altogether 6 doses were used and the relationship between inducibility and reactivity on the one hand and the fraction used on the other is illustrated in Figs. 3 and 4. Six weeks after the last tolerogenic dose the animals were immunized with 50 mg irradiated cell suspension. After another 6 weeks experimental mice and controls were challenged. Using the nuclear and microsomal fraction corresponding to 1 g of tumour given six times, tolerance was induced in a high percentage of animals. Non-reactivity was tested by an accelerated tumour growth in experimental animals compared with the controls, and by the inability of serum and immune cells from experimental animals to influence tumour growth in control mice. Using spleen colony formation assay AXELRAD (1963) found that mice of the AKR strain were tolerant to TSTA of Gross lymphoma (the virus of Gross lymphoma is endemic in AKR mice). He demonstrated further that C3H mice later showed reduced reactivity towards grafts of Gross lymphoma cells when inoculated with Gross virus as newborns (AXELRAD 1963, 1965).

Tumours induced by Gross virus, for example, in the C3H strain of mice were shown to contain TSTA (KLEIN et al., 1962). It was therefore of interest to find out whether spontaneous leukaemia of the AKR strain for which the Gross virus is responsible, also contains TSTA. GORER's method of allogeneic in vivo absorbed antiserum, or immunization of AKR strain mice against their own leukaemia was used for the detection of antigen. Allogeneic antisera were also tested for their cytotoxic activity using SCHREK's method. These antisera were absorbed repeatedly with an excess of normal AKR tissue from young animals. Both the in vitro cytotoxic test and the in vivo inhibition test showed that AKR leukaemia contained a specific antigen absent from normal AKR tissues, but failed to induce a detectable degree of resistance against leukaemia in AKR strain mice. This means that although AKR leukaemia contains TSTA, mice of the AKR strain are not capable of immunological reactions to this antigen. However, spontaneous leukaemia occurs in as much as 90% of female mice of the strain used. The virus causing leukaemia is transferred via placenta and probably through milk (METCALF, 1962). The most feasible explanation of the aforementioned results seems to us to be that mice of the AKR strain are naturally tolerant to TSTA of the leukaemia. Of these, almost all had an opportunity to meet the Gross virus and the tumour induced by it in the perinatal period, and thus natural tolerance was produced.

Analogous results in support of natural tolerance to AKR leukaemia were reported by WAHREN (1964, 1966). She found that AKR mice did not possess specific cytotoxic antibodies against AKR leukaemia. Antibodies, if ever found, were at low titre. The reaction of the transplantation type was practically indetectable.

KLEIN and KLEIN (1965) studied the reactivity of mice injected with homogenates of Moloney leukaemia, when newborn. Such mice showed a deficient or prolonged antibody response, as measured by an indirect fluorescence test. There was a correlation between antibody formation and the length of the preleukaemic, latent period.

HABEL (1962) found that adult mice develop resistance against tumours induced by polyoma virus as early as three days after virus inoculation, whereas in neonatal mice resistance is rarely detectable before the 24th post-injection day.

Recently, a number of very important works on immunology of spontaneous tumours of the C3H strain were published by WEISS et al. (1964), ATTIA et al. (1965), LAVRIN et al. (1966 a, b), BLAIR and WEISS (1966), MORTON (1964) and MORTON et al. (1965). In these experiments, both normal C3H mice and C3Hf mice were used; C3Hf mice are genetically and antigenically identical with C3H mice but free of oncogenic virus (free-f) and therefore no spontaneous mammary carcinomas develop in them. C3Hf mice were found to be resistant to spontaneous carcinomas, while C3H mice were not. Only tumour tissues could be used for preimmunization, because normal tissues from healthy mice had no effect on growth of C3H tumours. Resistance was accompanied by a distinct enlargement of the regional lymph nodes. Immune cells from these nodes and spleen were capable of adoptive transfer of immunity. One of the possible explanations is that the virus is endemic and induces natural tolerance in C3H mice that have a high incidence of mammary carcinomas. The aforementioned authors concentrated their attention on the question of the earliest appearance of the antigen specific for these spontaneous tumours. In the first place, they tried to find out whether this specific antigen may already be expressed in the preneoplastic hyperplastic alveolar nodules occurring in both C3H and C3Hf mice. The C3Hf mice were implanted with nodular tissues and after some time were tested with mammary tumour for immunity. The control animals were subjected to shame surgical procedure or were implanted with normal mammary tissues obtained from C3Hf donors. Both normal mammary tissues and alveolar nodules of C3Hf origin grew well in C3Hf recipients, did not produce an increased resistance to any of the two mammary tumours outgrowing form C3Hf. On the other hand, the nodular tissues were accompanied by clear signs of the transplantation reaction and usually did not take. Moreover, most of the C3Hf mice injected with nodular tissues in adult life proved to be resistant to subsequent challenge with spontaneous mammary carcinomas originating from these nodules. The results obtained can be best explained by assuming that the C3H nodular tissues and mammary carcinomas share an antigen which is absent in C3Hf animals. This antigenicity suggests that either a cellular antigen common to both the neoplastic and preneoplastic state of the mammary parenchyma (organ antigen?) or a viral antigen or virus-induced antigen might be present. Support for the presence of viral or virus-induced antigen was provided by MORTON (1964), who found that F_1 hybrids infected with milk antigen, when newborn, were less resistant to mammary carcinomas than F_1 hybrids suckled by the mother from a resistant strain. LAVRIN et al. (1966) infected neonatal C3Hf mice with MTV (mammary tumour virus) by foster-nursing on a C3H mother. Such animals were rendered non-reactive to growth of nodular tissues. Control experiments confirmed the specific suppression of immune reactions towards antigens of mammary tumours — tolerant mice were fully reactive towards all the other antigens tested. Further experiments were concentrated on the antigenicity of MTV virus, its antigenic similarity with the B-particles and the possible existence of NIV (nodule inducing virus) with low oncogenic activity which is also present in C3Hf mice (LAVRIN, 1966; LAVRIN, in press).

Immunological Enhancement in Relation to TSTA

As early as in the beginning of the century, FLEXNER and JOBLING (1910) found that the growth of inoculum of the same tumour was accelerated in rats pre-immunized with heat-inactivated tumour cells as compared with the controls. This phenomenon was later studied in detail in interstrain relationships of inbred mice. It has been found that it can be induced by preimmunization with frozen tumour tissues (XYZ factor — CASEY, 1949), lyophilized tissues (KALISS and SPAIN, 1952) and, in some instance, with intact tissues. This phenomenon has been called immunological enhancement, and although its main symptom is an acceleration of tumour growth, it is a specific immune, active response. Immunological enhancement can be transferred by antiserum, allogeneic antiserum being more effective than the heterologous one. A number of theories were formulated regarding the mechanism of immunological enhancement, as has been discussed in detail by KALISS (a review is given by KALISS, 1958, 1965, in Snell's paper, 1960). A very feasible explanation was presented by MÖLLER on the basis of his own experiments (MÖLLER, 1963 a, b, c) and the results described in the aforementioned papers. According to him, antibodies inhibit the formation of immune response and at the same time protect the tumour cells against destruction by immune cells. This protection is effected by coating with antibody all antigenic determinants on the surface of cells in which the tumour cells differ and thanks to which they may be destroyed by immune cells. In the syngeneic systems, the TSTA is the only antigenic difference between the host and tumour. If MÖLLER's concept is correct, and enhancement occurs when all antigenic receptors are coated with specific antibody, then immunological enhancement against TSTA should be possible. Acceleration of tumour growth after active immunization has repeatedly been observed in the syngeneic system (CASEY and GUNN, 1952; MIROFF et al., 1955), but convincing evidence has not been provided that enhancement as a specific immunological phenomenon, i. e. transfer by immune serum, was really involved. Since we also observed an accelerated tumour growth after active immunization in some experiments, attention was directed on the circumstances in which immunological enhancement or immunological tolerance might be responsible for acceleration (BUBENÍK and KOLDOVSKÝ, 1964, 1965). For immunization, either tumour suspensions irradiated with a dose of 20,000 r (methylcholanthrene-induced tumours) or ligature of subcutaneously or intracutaneously growing tumours were used. Irradiated suspensions were given in two doses — either 30 mg wet weight tumour (so-called small dose) or 300 mg (so-called large dose). Different schemes of immunization were employed as given for individual experiments. The state of immunity was estimated both by direct testing of immunized animals and especially by determining the capacity of their serum and immune cells to transfer immunity to the particular tumour. Adoptive transfer was carried out with lymph node cells in a ratio of 500 immune cells per tumour cell, and this mixture was incubated for 30 minutes and thereafter injected into untreated mice. Serum was

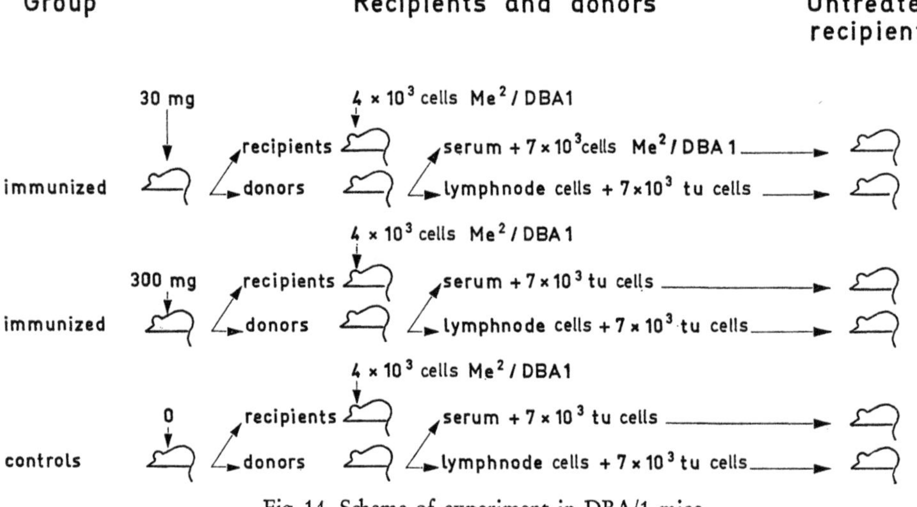

Fig. 14. Scheme of experiment in DBA/1 mice

administered intraperitoneally in two doses of 0.02 and 0.1 ml/mouse to untreated animals. Sixty minutes later, tumour cells mixed with aliquots of serum were inoculated. The same doses of antiserum were then given 3—4 times at intervals of three days. Two schemes of experiment will be given for illustration. The first scheme (Fig. 14) represents the experiment in which the effect of two doses on the nature of immune response was compared, a similar second experiment illustrates the effect of preimmunization with viable tumour (ligature of a growing tumour). Similar schemes were used in all experiments, but the results need not be given in detail. The following correlations were revealed. Lymph node cells from mice immunized with a small dose of irradiated cells, or by ligature of a growing tumour transferred mainly resistance. Immunological enhancement was also observed with tumour MC 2 in the DBA/1 strain. In this system, immunological enhancement was consistently obtained after adoptive transfer. The most likely explanation is that immune cells continue in producing enhancing antibodies and coat the tumour cells either during in vitro incubation or after injection into the recipient. MITCHISON and DUBE (1955) reported the transfer of enhancing antibodies by means of immune cells even in the allogeneic system (H-2 locus difference). McKHANN, however,

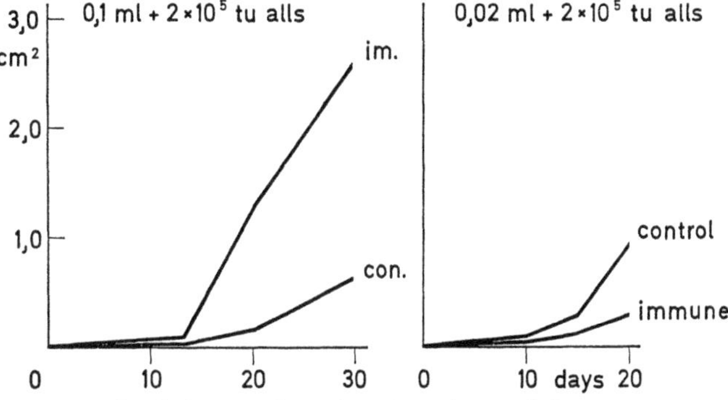

Fig. 15. The different effect of various doses of the same serum

failed to transfer enhancement by spleen cells with the difference in antigens controlled by the H-3 locus (McKHANN, 1962). In the same system, large immunizing doses resulted in production of non-reactive cells. Non-reactivity following large doses was also observed with the other tumours used. Serum from animals immunized with small doses transferred either partial resistance or enhancement. The result depended on the detection system used and the dose af antiserum. Essentially, larger doses — 0.1 ml — produced greater enhancement than smaller doses (0.02 ml) of antiserum (Fig. 15). Sometimes small doses were found to cause retardation of tumour growth (Fig. 16), while large doses were ineffective. It is difficult to explain, not to say to predict, why sometimes enhancement and sometimes resistance are transferred by serum. Either one kind of antibody is responsible for enhancement, and then only the proportion of antibody molecules and of determinant antigenic groups on the surface of cells is of decisive importance. Or, there may be two kinds of antibody, the one being responsible for enhancement, and the other for the retarding (cytotoxic?) effect. It can be assumed that in the former case larger doses (they were not used in the experiments described) may have direct cytotoxic effects on tumour cells. Medium doses (e. g. 0.1 ml $\pm 7 \cdot 10^3$ tumour cells) may coat all the determinant groups,

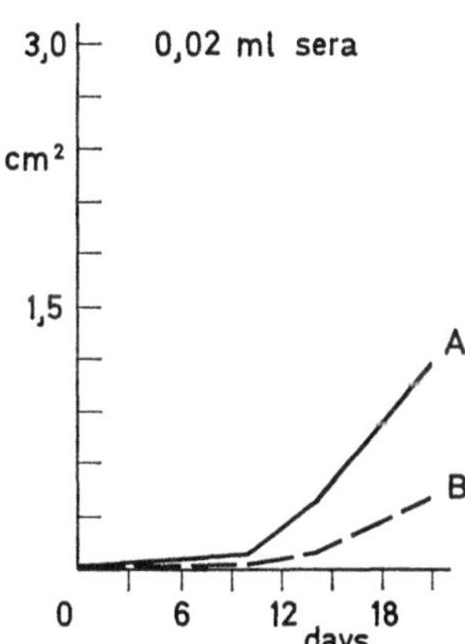

Fig. 16. Passive transfer of serum from DBA/2 mice immunized by rejection of tumour MC2/ DBA 2 after ligature. Curve A — untreated controls. Curve B — experimental group. 5 males per group

and enhancement occurs. Small doses may not be sufficient to obtain a full coating effect, but damage the tumour cells, and the growth is retarded. The possibility of an opsonin-like phenomenon cannot be excluded when growth is retarded in the whole body. Finally, a dose may exist which shows no effect of serum even though the serum contains antibody — the concentration of antibody is inadequate.

The second possibility suggesting the existence of two kinds of antibody has not
yet been confirmed experimentally. This question will be discussed in connection
with the role of 7S and 19S antibody. Theoretically, it can be assumed that
antibody responsible for retardation is analogous to cytotoxic antibody and
enhancing antibody is analogous to strongly avid blocking antibody. At one
time it has been believed that there might be two different kinds of antigen —
the one nuclear responsible for resistance and the other cytoplasmic responsible for

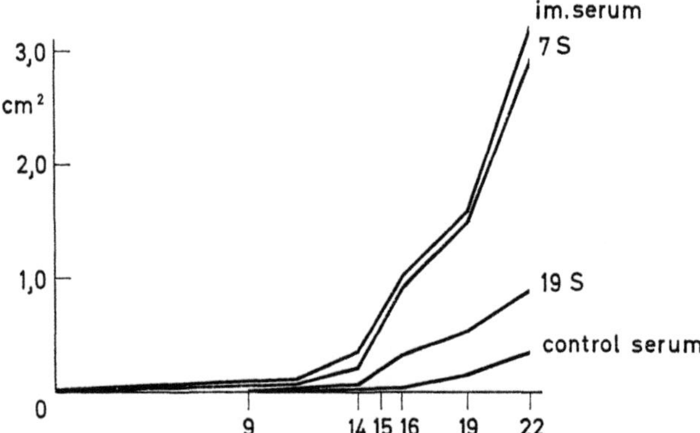

Fig. 17. The influence of immune serum and its fractions on the growth of tumour Mc2/DBA 1

enhancement. It is now generally accepted that the antigen(s) on the surface of cells
and not two kinds of antigen are involved. Analogous results in a similar experimental system of methylcholanthrene-induced tumours were reported by MÖLLER.
He used three tumours and observed a significant retardation of growth in two cases
and acceleration in one case after transfer by serum (MÖLLER, 1964).

Further experiments were centered on the question of the conditions in which
immunological enhancement occurs (BUBENÍK and KOLDOVSKÝ, 1965). The temporal
relations between enhancement and resistance were surprising in the syngeneic system
— it was precisely the reverse of what has been observed in the allogeneic system.
In the syngeneic system, the development of resistance (by the 6—7th week) followed
enhancement (by the 3rd—5th week). In the allogeneic system, KALISS (1956) observed that resistance was detectable already in the first weak after immunization,
then a decline in resistance was obvious and enhancement was usually not apparent
before the 4th week. KALISS found that the secondary graft of the same tumour
could be rejected by an intense immune reaction while the primary graft was enhanced. Thus, also in the allogeneic system enhancement may be followed by resistance (KALISS, 1962).

Attempts were made to define the molecular characteristics of serum factors
responsible for enhancement (BUBENÍK et al., 1965) or resistance. Mouse sera were
fractionated on a Sephadex G-200 column. A typical three-peak curve was obtained.
The peaks corresponded to the sedimentation constants of 19S, 7S and 4S respectively. Two kinds of immune sera were used in the experiments: the one, in the
given proportion of serum and tumour cells, caused retardation of tumour growth
(C57BL strain), and the other produced enhancement (DBA/1, DBA/2 strain).
Results with both these kinds of serum are illustrated in Fig. 17 and 18, and dia-

grammatically represented in Fig. 19. The activity of immune serum is localized in the gamma-globulin fraction. In serum, which as a whole shows inhibitory effects, the two immune fractions 7S and 19S cause retardation, the 19S fraction being

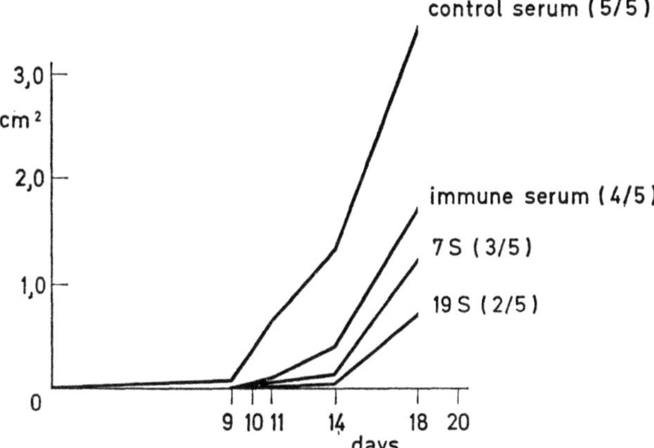

Fig. 18. The influence of immune serum and its fractions on the growth of tumour Mc1/C57BL. Ratio 0,02 ml sera mixed with 2×10^4 tumour cells per mouse

more effective than 7S. In serum, which as a whole produces enhancement, the two components also lead to enhancement, the 7S fraction being more effective in accelerating the tumour growth than the 19S fraction. For example, DIXON (1965)

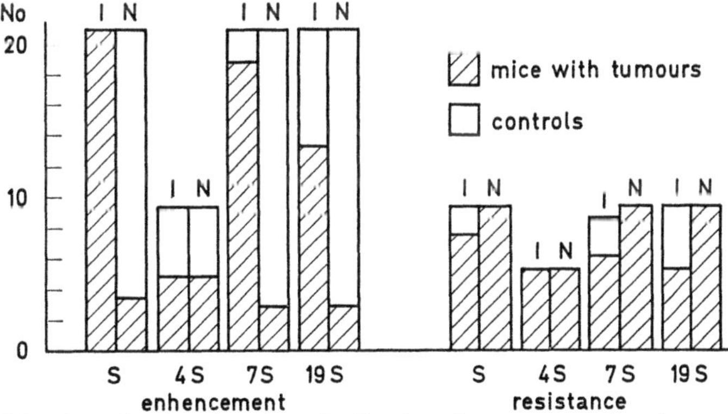

Fig. 19. Participation of 7 S and 19 S antibodies in enhancement and resistance to methyl-cholantrene-induced tumours. Cumulative data of 6 experiments. Controls — No: number of mice in the group. I — immune serum-fractions. N — normal serum-fractions. S — whole serum, 4 S, 7 S, 19 S-serum-fractions. The same controls were used for 7 S and 19 S-fraction — a mixture of whole serum and 7 S and 19 S were used for incubation with the tumour cells. The difference between the incidence of tumours in the experimental and control group (whole serum) is not significant

found that the 19S fraction from a heterologous antiserum was more effective than the 7S fraction in producing experimental nephritis. On the other hand, FINKELSTEIN and UHR (1964) reported that 7S antibody is more effective than 19S antibody in inhibiting antibody response since serum antibody formation may act as a "feedback" mechanism. On the basis of data obtained in our experiments it is impossible to decide whether the difference between the two fractions is due to the presence of antibodies of different specificity to a given antigen, or to a different avidity of antibodies, or to the different proportions of the particular antibody in the composition of 7S and 19S. The notion that 19S antibodies can inhibit more actively the host's resistance on the basis of antibody formation feed-back (and thus cause enhancement) is in agreement with the data in the literature.

Tumour Growth and Development of Immunity

The possibility of specific suppression of immune resistance against the tumour has been discussed in the previous two sections. From the theoretical and practical point of view, it is important to know the extent to which the tumour growth may interfere with immune reactions of the host organism, and how external non-specific influences may affect the tumour growth. These questions have been the subject of a number of lengthy reviews, from the point of view of both experimental tumours and clinical observations. It is neither possible nor feasible to give a comprehensive review here. I have, therefore, concentrated on certain aspects that seem of special relevance to the subject in hand. A number of factors have already been discussed in the section on immunity and carcinogenesis.

The same effects that generally influence immune reactions, may be involved in immunity directed against TSTA and thus play a role in tumour growth. Inbred strains of mice genetically differ, e. g. in their immunological reactivity (FINK and QUINN, 1953). It can be assumed that similar factors are also involved in resistance to the tumour. The F_1 hybrids of two mouse strains are not only more viable, but also have a better capacity for immunological reactivity against the tumour (KOLDOVSKÝ and BUBENÍK, 1963). The reaction against the tumour is altered as immunological reactivity changes with the age of animals (TELLER et al., 1954). The significance of the level of properdin for the occurrence and development of tumours could not be clearly confirmed (ORAVEC, 1964). Just as the mode and site of antigen injection is important for the development of immunity, the site of injection, the way in which the tumour grows and in which it may stimulate the immunological apparatus of the host is of special importance for the development of immunity directed against the tumour. The tumour is, however, also capable of growing against immunity, and this phenomenon was consistently observed even if immunity was directed against strong transplantation antigens controlled by the H-2 locus. Influences adverse to the course of infectious diseases, such as exhaustion, non-physiological stress, a further intercurrent disease, may also show adverse effects on the resistance to the tumour. Cortisone treatment not only increases the takes of tumours so that the heterologous barriers may be overcome (TOOLAN, 1957), but also accelerates tumour growth and increases its metastasizing ability. Similarly, wholebody irradiation or treatment with cytostatics stimulates the tumour growth. On the other hand, all treatments non-specifically stimulating the host defence mechanisms may cause delay in tumour growth. For example, the efficacy of immunization against TSTA may be increased by the addition of FREUND's adjuvant (FINK et al., 1955). The addition of BCG alone may also influence the tumour growth and it is surprising to see how long a non-specific stimulation persists (OLD and CLARENCE, 1959). From this point of view, the intercurrent milder diseases might sometimes have beneficial effects as non-specific stimulants. A number of clinical observations and the experiment of ZEIDMAN and BUSS (1954) on the behaviour of V2 carcinoma metastasizing into the lymphatic vessels of the rabbit show how long the local barrier of regional lymph nodes may prevent further dissemination of tumour cells in the host. The tumour grew in the system closest to regional lymph nodes and it took at least 3 weeks and usually more before it spread to a further node. The activation of the RES may still increase the defence mechanisms against metastasizing tumours. YAMAGUCHI et al. (1965) found that the tumour injected into the tail of the mouse metastasized into the draining nodes in 46.4% of cases when the tail was amputated 10 days after tumour inoculation. When animals were previously stimulated with typhoid vaccine, the percentage of metastases fell to 16.1. Conversely, the reduction of reactivity of the RES by prednisol resulted in the rise to 58.3%.

Numerous studies dealt with the question whether the growing tumour is capable of non-specifically suppressing immune reactions towards other antigens. And, if this is so, whether there is any relationship between the histological type of tumour and the degree of its development. It should be emphasized that in these experiments the type of antigen and the species of the host are of particular importance. A good example is the difference in the effect of methylcholanthrene on immune reactions (no effect on serum antibody response in rabbits, great effects on transplantation immunity in mice), as has been mentioned in the previous section. ISHIBASHI (1965) failed to demonstrate the suppression of immune antibody response in animals bearing tumours. This suppression escaped detection even though the tumour was well developed. On the other hand, the delayed type reaction was significantly weaker in tumour bearers, as has been shown by skin tbc reactions and skin graft survival. This finding is very important from the point of view of immunity directed against a weak TSTA. MATSUOKA (1965) did not find a changed primary antibody response in animals bearing tumours, but sometimes observed reduction of the secondary response. Of the clinical tumours, tumours of the RES — leukaemias, lymphomas and reticulosarcomas received greatest attention. The relevant literature has been reviewed, for example, by LIBÁNSKÝ (1965). It seems to be proved that antibody response to bacterial antigens is not suppressed in any of the above types of tumour, except for reticuloses in children. Most of these studies are hampered by the interference of chemotherapy with immune reactivity of the host. As shown by CROCH et al. (1965) chemotherapy displayed no influence on the phagocytic activity of the RES (CROCH et al., 1965), but the majority of patients with leukaemia had a decreased phagocytic activity. Finally, clinical studies directed attention to comparison of the reactivity of tumour-bearing patients and patients without tumour to tuberculin. Although contradictory results were obtained, the tuberculin reaction seems to be suppressed in tumour-bearing patients (BEK et al., in press).

Theoretical and Practical Possibilities of the Presence of Transplantation Immunity against Tumours in Man

The existence of TSTA has now been demonstrated in a considerable variety of tumours of experimental animals. The ability of the host organism to recognize the TSTA as foreign and to react against it by transplantation resistance is also very important. From the immunobiological point of view, man does not represent an exception in this respect, and thus it can be assumed that some of the human tumours also possess TSTA and that the human organism is capable of reacting by the transplantation reaction. This possibility has been suggested by a large body of follow-up data from experimental and clinical investigations, but critical evidence for the existence of TSTA in human tumours, as known, for example, for virus-induced animal tumours, is not yet available.

Indirect Evidence

Some clinical observations (spontaneous regression, infiltration by immune cells, presence of malignant cells without progressive tumour growth), not giving direct evidence of the immune mechanisms of the patients can nevertheless best be explained on the basis of such defence reactions. SMITH et al. (1958) studied the relationship between cytological detection of tumour cells in an operation wound and a number of other factors. No correlation was found between the presence of cancer cells and the type of operation, degree of tumour dedifferentiation, size of the primary tumour and the presence of metastatic nodes. Progressive tumour growth started in 53% of patients showing cancer cells in the operation wound. In some patients residual malignant cells were probably destroyed after the operation. Nevertheless, the finding of malignant cells is associated with an unfavourable prognosis, because progressive growth was observed in only 29% of patients in which no such cells were found. Some tumours remain clinically silent for years, sometimes throughout the whole life of the patient. HIRST and BERGMAN (1954) reported that at autopsy the carcinoma of the prostate could be found 4 to 10 times as frequently as revealed by the clinical diagnosis. As early as 1934 POOL and DUNLOP demonstrated the presence of malignant cells in blood much more frequently than expected by the occurrence of metastases. This observation was later confirmed by ENGELL (1959). Tumour cells were found not only in the blood, but also in the lymph (WATME et al., 1959), and the pleural fluid (SPJUT, 1958) although metastases did not develop in all cases.

In some mammary carcinomas, BERG (1959) observed inflammatory reactions as judged by the presence of plasma cells. Inflammatory reactions have a favourable prognosis. The lymphocytic and easinophilic infiltration also appeared to be of a favourable prognostic value with cancer of the stomach (YOON, 1959). Such morphological changes were shown to be really manifestations of the defence mechanisms of the host organism and not reactions against an intercurrent infection by GRACE and DAO (1958). In their experiments skin tests with antigen prepared from the patient's own tumour were positive only when inflammatory reactions were also present. According to GRAHAM and GRAHAM (1955) antibodies in serum of patients with tumour disease, demonstrable by complement fixation, had a favourable prognosis. They observed such antibodies in 12 out of 48 patients with gynaecological carcinomas.

EVERSON and COLE (1959) and SMITHERS (1964) gave a review of verified cases of spontaeous regression of human neoplasma. EVERSON and COLE summarize in a table 112 cases of spontaneous regression including 7 types of malignant tumours which are most frequently reported to regress spontaneously. These are embryonic tumours in children, the chorioepithelioma, adenocarcinomas of the kidney, malignant melanomas, soft tissue sarcomas, carcinomas of the bladder, carcinomas of the breast. SMITHERS proposes to add carcinomas of the ovary to these seven tumours. It is of interest that in two cases of inoperable embryonic tumours in children COLEY's toxin has been applied which could non-specifically stimulate the immune apparatus of the host organism. It should be taken into account that the majority of the above tumours are hormone-dependent. SMITH and STEHLIN (1965) studied in detail spontaneous regression of primary malignant melanomas and of their regional metastases. The occurrence of metastatic foci without the finding of the primary tumour may best account for spontaneous regression of the primary tumour. Regression of the primary tumour, however, does not mean that metastasizing tumours are less malignant.

CUTLER et al. (1966) investigated the relationship between sinus histiocytic reactivity of lymph nodes and the survival of a breast carcinoma and at the same time gave a review of the earlier publications pertaining to similar relationships.

The types of indirect evidence just outlined are, however, less important than experiments and observations revealing that an "autoimmune disease" of the tumour may really sometimes occur even in man. In a number of his works GRACE paid attention to the "take" of autologous tumour cells in relation to skin reactions with purified antigen. He found that the take of primary tumours was very low when patients gave positive skin reactions (GRACE, 1964; GRACE and KONDO, 1958). A defence mechanism seems to exist which does not allow even the implantation metastases to grow progressively. Similar results with the fate of tumour autografts were obtained by KOIKE et al. (1963). They studied the behaviour of autografts and of heterologous and allogeneic tumour grafts. In numerous works SOUTHAM studied the reactivity of patients and the fate of tumours as well as the possibility of detecting immune reactions against tumours in clinical practice using the methods of transplantation resistance. In autotransplantation experiments he found (SOUTHAM, 1964) that the tumour did not usually grow until 10^8 cells were inoculated, whereas the doses 1—2 logarithms lower grew in half the patients under study. This observation can be explained in two ways — either the ability for growth is the result of the intrinsic growth potential of those cancer cells, or the host is capable of inhibiting the growth of transplanted cells. The host might then also be able to inhibit the naturally disseminated cancer cells. The growth potential of human cancer cells can be studied either in tissue culture or on heterologous hosts with depressed immune reactions. Some of the cancer cells may be shown to have a greater growth potential than they display in autotransplantation. Studies of host defence mechanisms against cancer show that the ability to form antibodies is practically normal, but positive skin reaction to dinitrofluorobenzene is reduced. The most impressive defect of the patient's defence mechanisms is seen by SOUTHAM in reduced responsiveness to transplants. He studied this reactivity by inoculating human cancer cells cultivated in vitro in many experiments. Such cells were shown to grow for 3—4 weeks or sometimes longer before the signs of regression appeared in most of the patients with advanced cancer. The prolonged survival of tumour homografts is not confined to patients with tumours of the reticulo-endothelial system or those treated with cytostatics (immunosuppressive drugs). The antigenicity of these tumour cells was confirmed in healthy volunteers, who had rejected the transplants very rapidly. In more than 200 cancer patients the degree of their inability to react against transplanted tumours has been found to be in correlation with the degree of tumour development. Using volunteers immunized with tumour cell lines and absorption of their sera SOUTHAM demonstrated that the tumour cells contained the antigen(s) absent in normal human tissues. In his view, the inability to react against tumour allografts is attributable to the reduction of the patient's reactivity rather than to its complete suppression. According to LEVIN et al. (1964) it is not directly dependent on the degree of the general debility caused by the tumour disease.

Of considerable interest are the experiments of SOUTHAM (1965 a, b) regarding the effect of admixture of autologous lymphoid cells on the growth of tumour auto-transplants ("adoptive transfer of immunity"). These experiments show the extent to which the rejection of metastases may be mediated by immune, cellular reactions of the host's own organism. In the section on Mechanisms of antitumour immunity it has been emphasized that an excess of immune cells is required for the destruction of tumour cells. Hence, if a spontaneous metastasis in the patient's body is not soon surrounded by an excess of immune, sensitized cells, it can grow progressively, in the reverse case it may be destroyed. SOUTHAM added 10×10^6 lymphocytes and leucocytes prepared from peripheral blood to tumour autotransplant. The number of tumour cells varied from 10,000 to 100,000,000. In half the patients under study the growth of autotransplanted tumour cells was inhibited, as a result of the admixture of leucocytes and lymphocytes. Autologous plasma was shown to have a lesser inhibitory effect. Allogeneic leucocytes showed greater variations — growth was inhibited in 6 cases and in 3 cases the tumour autotransplant was enhanced.

The study of FINNEY et al. (1960) regarding the possible immunotherapy of human tumour disease is of particular interest. They studied two groups of patients with advanced malignant disease. The first group of 5 patients had undergone X-ray therapy. Of these, 3 patients contained detectable antibodies, and some metastatic nodes regressed. The second group of patients were immunized with antigen prepared from their own tumours in FREUND's adjuvant. Marked inflammatory reactions at the tumour site were noted. A gamma-globulin fraction was prepared from serum and was injected directly into the metastatic subcutaneous cancer lesions. This was followed by softening and shrinkage in size of metastases, but the cure was impossible by this means.

The effect of an autogenous tumour vaccine on the course of tumour disease and the antigenicity of this vaccine was studied by M. ASWAQ (1964) using passive skin anaphylaxy (PCA test) in guinea-pigs. For PCA tests he used serum from the patients after immunization. Sera from all vaccinated patients showed positive PCA, whereas control sera gave negative results. Positive sera did not react with antigen from normal tissues. The vaccines, however, failed to provide sufficient benefit to the vaccinated patients to recommend their use in treatment.

In 1953—1954 GORODILOVA (1965) vaccinated 32 female patients with mammary tumours after surgical removal and irradiation. Another group of 34 patients with clinically comparable tumours were given conventional treatment. Autolysed tumour tissues prepared from a pool of various mammary carcinomas was used for immunization, autologous tissue was never used. Immunization was performed 5 times at intervals of 5—7 days. Allergic reactions were noted in some patients.

13 vaccinated and 23 non-vaccinated patients were dead within 5 years. 18 vaccinated patients and only 11 non-vaccinated patients survive for more than 10 years. The relationship between the occurrence of allergic reactions and the length of survival was surprising. All patients (10) with strong allergic reactions had died within $2^1/_2$ years, the 13 patients without any reactions were alive at the time of publication, more than 10 years after vaccination.

HUGHES and LYTTON (1964) used subcellular material prepared by disintegrating the cells by sonication and differential centrifugation for a follow-up of the patient's reactivity by means of skin tests. Of the 33 patients examined, 5 gave positive reactions.

Vaccination with a suspension of human HeLa cells to which COLEY's toxin is added (a mixture of toxin of Streptococcus A seratia marcescens) was proposed by PELNER and RHOADES (1963) for human beings in which the tumour has not yet been established. This miture has to be suspended in FREUND's adjuvant and injected intracutaneously. As has been emphasized by the authors, this kind of vaccination is based on the assumption of a common tumour antigen. This possibility has been excluded for TSTA of experimental animal tumours, and it is unlikely that it may hold for human tumours.

MAKARI (1965) prepared a polysaccharide substance from the mitochondrial fraction of tumour cells and studied its antigenicity and the reactivity of patients by means of intracutaneous tests. In the years 1958—1965, altogether 858 persons were tested, 298 being cancer patients. Tests were positive in 83% of localized tumours, in 55.3% of tumours extended locally and in 20.9% of tumours metastasizing into distant organs. In cancer patients, regarded as cured after 5 years, skin tests were negative in all 12 cases. It can be considered that the reactivity of the patient is impaired as the tumour develops, and conversely, the malignant disease progresses as the reactivity decreases.

WIMER (1965) tried to influence the granulocytic leukaemia in a 31-year-old man with bone marrow and leucocytes from his parents. Together with leucocytes androgens were administered. Progressive improvement was observed after the injection of leucocytes, but an intercurrent disease (sinusitis) disturbed a full recovery of the patient.

In connection with the possibility of using patient's autologous lymphocytes, a study of ROBINSON and HOCHMAN (1966) should be remembered. The showed that lymphocytes from cancer patients elicited weaker skin reactions in the recipient than did lymphocytes from healthy persons. They believed the lymphocytes from cancer patients were antigenically deficient. Allogeneic spleen cells were used by WOODRUFF and NOLAN (1963), who observed a definite clinical improvement. The effects of heterologous sheep lymphocytes on benzpyrene-induced tumours in rats were investigated by ALEXANDER et al. (1966), who found that primary fibrosarcomas were inhibited by lymphocytes from the efferent duct lymphonode of immunized sheep. They take the view that heterologous lymphocytes may strengthen the immune reactions of their own hosts. The extent to which such procedures might be utilized in clinical practice is still a subject of controversy.

Interest has recently developed in BURKITT's tumour which is suspected to be of virogenic origin. Using membrane fluorescence, KLEIN et al. (1966) studied the reaction of the patient with both normal and tumour cells. They obtained a definite, though not conclusive, evidence that the Burkitt sarcoma contained tumour specific antigen. Of interest is the finding that immune responses were more pronounced in patients showing a favourable response to chemotherapy. In the light of preliminary results (obtained in a relatively small number of cases) the reactivity of patients with BURKITT's lymphoma seems to be specifically reduced against this tumour (KOLDOVSKÝ et al., 1966).

The Possibility of the Presence of Organ Specific Antigen in Cancer Tissues

A variety of organs contain specific antigens, but autoimmune reactions against them are rare. The original organ may be protected against autoimmune disease by the same mechanisms that are not yet known but prevent the development of auto-immunity against organ specific antigens in healthy persons. From this point of view, the so-called GRAWITZ's tumour in the stage of lung metastases is of particular interest. Spontaneous regression of lung metastases has been consistently observed after the primary tumour had been excised (e. g. ARCOMONE et al., 1958; KOLÁR et al., 1961). We studied in detail 5 patients after surgical removal of the primary tumour (JAKOUBKOVÁ et al., 1965) and confirmed the data reported in the literature that radical removal is also indicated for the stage of lung metastases. However, it should be emphasized that with this tumour an atypical behaviour of distant metastases is specific only for the metastases in the lungs. As known from the literature and as we could also see in other patients, removal of the primary tumour had no effect on bone and brain metastases. Theoretically, the reaction of lung metastases might best be explained on the immunological basis. After removal of the primary tumour the host organism will no longer be flooded with excess of antigen and his defence mechanisms may be non-specifically depressed. It should be recalled that the lungs as an organ consistently exposed to infectious stimuli from the external environment have relatively strong defence mechanisms. It can be presumed that the GRAWITZ's tumour possesses an organ specific antigen of the kidney which on stimulating the organism apart from the kidney, may induce immunity. It is of interest that a similar behaviour was noted with the lung metastases of a chorioepithelioma in which foreign (father) transplantation antigens can be presumed.

Similarly, organ-specific antigens might be present in tumours of the testis, the brain etc., but as far as is known from the literature, the presence of organ specific antigens has not been studied in human tumours of this type. Using absorption of rabbit antiserum and immunofluorescence JURAND and HIRAMOTO (1966) demonstrated in mouse rhabdomyosarcoma the presence of normal myosine cross-reacting not only with mouse but also with human myosine.

Chorioepithelioma

Chorioepithelioma takes an unusual place among human tumours because of its rarity and particularly because of its aetiology. This tumour originates from foetal tissues, i. e. from tissues genetically foreign to the organism [only the more frequently occurring placental chorioepithelioma (in females — after pregnancy) will be discussed] and hence is biologically an allograft (homograft) of tumour tissue. Since transplantation antigens are inherited dominantly, if not lost during malignant conversion, the chorioepithelioma should contain a number of transplantation antigens contributed by the father. Thus a comparably high frequency of spontaneous regression of this tumour, the success of chemotherapy and of specific immunotherapy can be explained.

If one goes over the whole problem in detail, the question is reversed, i. e. why a tumour homograft which is virtually the chorioepithelioma, grows progressively and is not rejected like other tumour homo(allo)grafts in human beings. In the first place, it is well known from experiments and from some clinical observations that the tumour is capable of growing even against immunity. Moreover, the transplantation reactivity against father antigens seems to be specifically inhibited after pregnancy. BREYER and BARRETT (1960) showed that allotransplantation immunity was reduced to a male possessing histocompatible antigens of the transplant. In this case, experiments involved transplantation of DBA/2 sarcoma on a BALB/c female which gave birth to offspring after having been mated to DBA/2 males. In similar experiments, WOODRUFF (1957) and MEDAWAR and SPARROW (1956) obtained negative results. Later on, BREYER and BARRETT (1961) extended their experiments to mating the BALB/c females with other males (differing at different antigens controlled by the H-2 locus). They used only one C3H-specific tumour (specific for C3H) which grew in 59% of females mated to C3H males and delivering the offspring, in less than 1% of females mated to syngeneic males and in none of the other females. The immune response was therefore specifically depressed. Similar results — tolerance induction — were obtained by PREHN (1960), who found that the degree of tolerance corresponded to the number of litters. Partial tolerance could also be induced by mating females to sterile males. PREHN discussed this question in relation to chorioepithelioma.

The discrepancy between the results of PREHN and those of BREYER and BARRETT on the one hand and of MEDAWAR and SPARROW on the other can be explained by the difference in antigenic dissimilarities employed. It is conceivable that tolerance towards strong transplantation antigens is difficult or impossible to induce. HAŠKOVÁ (1963) studied the antigenicity of the placenta according to its ability to elicit second set reaction towards skin grafts. The placenta manifest itself as antigenic or nonantigenic, according to whether a weak or strong antigenic difference is used.

The question of immunity and spontaneous regression of chorioepithelioma has been discussed in detail by BARDAWIL and TOY (1959). They gave a detailed review of the extensive literature on the possible use of immunotherapy and quoted SCHMAUCH from 1903 that inoperable cases of choriocarcinoma should be treated by means of specific antibodies.

ROBINSON et al. (1963) observed a surprisingly long survival of the husband's skin graft in a female patient with chorioepithelioma. The skin graft from a randomly selected donor was rejected normally in both cases, i. e. within 7 and 14 days respectively, the graft from the husband within 3 and 2 months respectively. Antibodies agglutinating the husband's leucocytes were not produced. CINADER et al. (1963) made attempts at specific immunotherapy of choriocarcinoma. They used both active (repeated administration of husband's leucocytes) and passive immunity (injection of rabbit antiserum against the husband's sperm). Both immune treatments resulted in an apparent reduction of hormone production and the disappearance of lung metastases. Mathé et al. (1964) studied immunologically 5 females patients with metastases of chorioepithelioma. The serum of two patients had leucoagglutinins in low titre against their husband's leucocytes, but in the other three patients the antibody titre was remarkably high. Four of these were given skin grafts from their husbands; the survival time approached the upper limit of the norm in patients with a high titre of leucoagglutinins, whereas a longer survival was noted in patients with a low antibody titre. The reaction to the second graft was also retarded.

We performed active immunization with husband's leucocytes in two cases of choriocarcinoma (Jakoubková et al., 1965), and observed the disappearance of lung metastases depending on the time of immunization in one case. The patient is now without evidence of disease at four years after treatment. The other patient showed only a transient, but objective (roentgenologically) shrinkage of the metastases. In this case, immunization was started at an infaust state when surgical treatment (repeated operations) and chemotherapy were no longer efficacious and the cancer continued to grow progressively until the patient had died. At the persent time, several patients with chorioepithelioma are being treated with chemotherapy and active immunization after the primary tumour has been excised. In one of these patients in which chemotherapy did not appear to offer a very promising prospect, HCG disappeared after specific active immunization and non-specific stimulation, and the patient is clinically negative. A similar course of the disease was observed in another case, but the remaining patients could not yet be evaluated at the present time.

Summary and Perspectives

TSTA has been convincingly demonstrated for a variety of experimental tumours of various aetiology — it is most markedly expressed in tumours induced by oncogenic viruses and carbohydrate carcinogens. The host organism is able to react against these antigens in the same manner as against other, normal weak transplantation antigens. Immune reactions are mediated by immunologically competent cells. Under certain circumstances, these reactions may be depressed on the basis of immunological tolerance or immunological enhancement. The reduction of antigenicity or adaptation of the tumour may also have adverse effects on these reactions.

Although clear evidence cannot as yet be provided for human cancer, as it has been obtained in experiments on animals, it is likely that at least some human tumours will contain TSTA and that immune reactions against TSTA will also be elicited in man. The demonstration of TSTA may be of diagnostic value, but may also make possible a sound approach to the problems of viral aetiology of human tumours (TSTA common to tumours induced by the same virus). Finally, it might be used for therapeutic purposes. At the present stage of knowledge, it is possible that immunotherapy as a useful adjunctive procedure may be of help in eliminating the residual tumour cells left behind by surgery, actinotherapy or chemotherapy, at least in some selected cases. It is anticipated that in the future vaccination with viral vaccines may yield significant benefit in cancer prophylaxis.

Acknowledgments

To say thank you to everyone involved in the writing of this paper would be literally impossible. However, I must express my gratitude to Prof. HASEK, who first initiated these experiments and has supported them very effectively. I would also like to thank Dr. SVOBODA and Dr. BUBENÍK. It was a pleasure to work together with them and to have them participate in our experiments. Last but not least, I am indebted to Mrs. ZAHOUROVA for her excellent technical help.

References

AHLSTRÖM, C. G.: Neoplasms in mammals induced by Rous chicken sarcoma material. Nat. Cancer Inst. Monogr. 17, 299 (1964).

ALEXANDER, P.: Biological methods against cancer. New Scientist 24, 884 (1964).

—, E. J. DELORME, J. G. HALL, and D. AUST: The effect of lymphoid cells from the lymph of specifically immunized sheep on the growth of primary sarcomata in rats. Lancet 1186, 1966.

— —, L. D. HAMILTON, and J. G. HALL: Effect of nucleic acids from immune lymphocytes on rats a sarcomata. Nature 213, 509 (1967).

ALGIRE, G. H., J. M. WEAVER, and R. T. PREHN: Studies on tissue homotransplantation in mice using diffusion chamber methods. Ann. N. Y. Acad. Sci. 64, 1009 (1957).

ANDERVONT, H. B.: The use of pure strain animals in studies on natural resistance to transplantable tumors. Pub. Hlth Rep. 82, 1885 (1937).

APPEL, C. A., B. AMESON, and J. H. PETTERS: Submitted for publication.

ARCAMONO, J. P., J. C. BARNETT, and J. J. BOTTORE: Spontaneous disappearence of pulmonary metastases following nephrectomy for hypernephroma. Amer. J. Surg. 96, 703 (1958).

ASWAQ, M.: Immunological response to autologous cancer vaccine. Arch. Surgery 89, 485 (1964).

AXELRAD, A. A.: Changes in resistance to the proliferation of isotransplanted Gross-virus induced lymphoma cells as measured with a spleen colony assay. Nature 199, 80 (1963).

— Antigenic behaviour of lymphoma cell population in mice as revealed by the spleen colony method. Progr. exp. Tumour Res. 6, 31 (1965).

—, and G. KLEIN: Differences in histocompatibility of primary tumor and its metastases. Transpl. Bull. 2, 100 (1956).

ATTIA, M. A.: Enhancement of a spontaneous tumor in the strain of origin following vaccination with a tumor membrane fraction. Proc. Amer. Ass. Cancer. Res. 4, 3 (1963).

—, K. B. DeOME, and D. W. WEIS: Immunology of spontaneous mammary carcinoma in mice. Resistance to a rapidly and slowly developing tumor. Cancer Res. 25, 451 (1965).

BALDWIN, R. W.: Immunity to methylcholantrene induced tumors in inbred rats following atrophy and regression of the implanted tumors. Brit. J. Cancer 9, 682 (1955).

BALL, J. K., N. R. SINCLAIR, and J. A. McCARTEE: Prolonged immunosuppresion and tumor induction by chemical carcinogen injected at birth. Science 152, 659 (1966).

BALNER, H., and H. DERSJANT: Neonatal thymectomy and tumor induction with methylcholantrene in mice. J. nat. Cancer Inst. 36, 513 (1966).

BARDAWIL, W. A., and B. L. TOY: The natural history of chorionepitheliom problems of immunity and spontaneous regression. Ann. N. Y. Acad. Sci. 80, 197 (1959).

BARRET, M. K., and M. K. DERRINGER: An induced adaptation in transplantable tumor of mice. J. nat. Cancer Inst. 11, 51 (1950).

— —, and W. H. HANSEN: Induced adaption of a tumor. Specificity of the change. J. nat. Cancer Inst. 14, 381 (1953).

BATCHELOR, J. R., and N. CHAPMAN: The influence of sex upon the antibody response an incompatible tumour. Immunol. 9, 553 (1965).

BAUER, H., u. W. SCHÄFER: Isolierung eines gruppenspezifischen Antigens aus dem Hühner-Myeloblastose-Virus (BAI Stamm A). Z. Naturforsch. 20 b, 815 (1965).

BENNET, B.: Phagocytosis of mouse tumor cells in vitro by various homologous and heterologous cells. J. Immunol. 95, 80, (1965).

—, J. L. OLD, and E. A. BOYSE: Opsonisation of cells by isoantibodies in vitro. Nature 198, 10 (1963).

— — The phygocytosis of tumor cells in vitro. Transplantation 2, 183 (1964).

BERG, J. W.: Inflammation and prognosis in breast cancer. A search for host resistance. Cancer 12, 714 (1959).

BESREDKA, A., et L. GROSS: De l'immunisation contre le sarcome de la souris par voie intracutanée. Ann. Inst. Pasteur 55491 (1935).

BIGGS, M. W., and J. E. EISELSTEIN: Diffusion chamber studies of allogeneic tumor immunity in mice. Cancer Res. 25, 1888 (1965).

BITTNER, J. J.: A review of genetic studies on the transplantation of tumors. J. Genetics 31, 471 (1935).

BORGES, P. R. F., and B. J. KVEDAR: A mutation producing resistance to several transplantable neoplasm in the C57BL mice. Cancer Res. 12, 19 (1952).

BREYER, E. J., and M. K. BARRET: Tolerance induced by parity in mice incompatible at the H-2 locus. J. nat. Cancer Inst. 27, 409 (1961).

BRONDZ, B. D.: Interaction of immune lymphocytes in vitro with normal and neoplastic tissue cells. Folia Biol. (Praha) 10, 164 (1964 a).

— Antibodies to the specific antigen of tumor cell membrane (in Russian). Vop. onkol. 10, 81 (1964 b).

BUBENÍK, J., B. ADAMCOVÁ, and P. KOLDOVSKÝ: A contribution of the antigenicity of spontaneous lymphoid AKR leukemia. Folia Biol. (Praha) 10, 293 (1964).

— — — Changes in the antigenicity of tumours passaged against immunoselective pressure. Proc. Symp. Genetic Variation in Somatic Cells, Prague 1965, 403.

— — — The dual effect of antibodies against sex-linked histocompatibility antigen. Folia Biol. (Praha) 12, 11 (1966).

—, and H. BAUER: Antigenic characteristics of the interaction between Rous sarcoma virus and mammalian cells. Virology 31, 489 (1967).

—, J. IVANYI, and P. KOLDOVSKÝ: Heterogenity of antitumor antibodies. Folia Biol. (Praha) 11, 240 (1965).

— — — Participation of 7 S and 19 S antibodies in enehěncement and resistance to methylcholanthrene induce tumors. Folia biol. (Praha) 11, 426 (1965).

—, P. KOLDOVSKÝ, J. SVOBODA, V. KLEMENT, and R. DVORÁK: Induction of tumours in mice with three variants of Rous sarcoma virus and studies on the immunobiology of these tumours. Folia biol. (Praha) 13, 29 (1967).

BURDICK, K. H., and W. HAWK.: Vitiligo in a case of vaccinia-virus treated melanoma. Cancer 17, 708 (1964).

CASEY A., L. GORDON, L. ROSS, and R. R. LAUGSTON: Selective XYZ factor in C57BL mammary carcinoma Eo 771. Proc. Soc. exp. Biol. Med. 72, 83 (1949).

CASEY, A. N., and J. GUNN: XYZ effect on strain of origin: Eo 771 carcinoma in C57BL/6 mice. Proc. Soc. exp. Biol. Med. 80, 610 (1952).

CHANG S., and W. H. HILDEMAN: Inheritance of susceptibility to polyoma virus in mice J. nat. Cancer Inst. 33, 303 (1964).

CINADER, B., M. A. HALEY, W. D. RIDER, and O. H. WARWICK: Immunotherapy of a patient with choriocarcinoma. Canad. med. Ass. J. 84, 306 (1961).

CLOUDMAN, A. M.: A genetic analysis of dissimilar carcinomata from the sam gland of individual mouse. Genetics 17, 468 (1922).

CLOWES, G. H. A.: Further evidence of immunity against cancer in mice after spontaneous recovery. Med. News 87, 968 (1905).

CREECH, H. J.: Immunological properties of conjugates prepared from proteins and isogametes of polynuclear aromatic hydrocarbons. Acta int. contre Cancer 6, 451 (1949).

— Chemical and immunobiological properties of carcinogeb-protein conjugates. Cancer Res. 12, 557 (1952).

CUDKOWICZ, G.: Evidence for immunisation of F_1 hybride mice against parental transplantation antigen. Proc. Soc. exp. Biol. Med. 107, 968 (1961).

CUDKOWICZ, G., and G. E. VE GOSGRO: Modified homologous disease following transplantation of parental bone marrow and recipient liver into irradiated F_1 mice. Transpl. Bull. 27, 90 (1961).

CUTLER, S. J., M. M. BLACK, G. H. FRIEDEL, R. A. VIDONE, and I. S. GOLDENBERG: Prognostic factors in cancer of the female breast. II. Reproducibility of histopathology classfication. Cancer 19, 75 (1966).

DAVIDOVSK, I., K. STERN, and L. SABERT: Immune response in mice and rats exposed to cancerogenesis. Proc. Amer. Ass. Cancer Res. 2, 102 (1956).

DAVIES, D. A. L.: H-2 histocompatibility antigens of the mouse. "Transplantation". Ciba Found. Symp. 45, (1962).

—, E. A. BOYSE, L. J. OLD, and E. STOCKERT: Mouse isoantigens: separation of soluble TL antigen from soluble H-2 antigen by column chromatography. J. exp. Med. 125, 549 (1967).

DAWE, C. J., L. W. LAW, and T. B. DUNN: Studies on parotid tumor agent in cultures of leukemic tissues of mice. J. nat. Cancer Inst. 23, 717 (1959).

DAY, E. D.: The immunochemistry of cancer. Thomas Springfield, Ill.: C.C.C. 1965.

DECKERS, C., and J. MAISIN: Etude comparative de la structure antigenique d'un hépatome transplantable et du foie chez le rat. Rev. belge. Path. 28, 477 (1961).

DEFENDI, V., and R. A. ROOSA: The role of the thymus in cancerogenesis The thymus. Wistar Inst. Symp. Monograph. No. 2., 1964, p. 121.

— — Effect of thymectomy on induction of tumors and on the transplantability of polyoma induced tumors. Cancer Res. 25, 300 (1965).

DEICHMAN, G. I., and T. E. KLUCHAREVA: Prevention of tumor induction in SV40 infected hamsters. J. nat. Cancer Inst. 32, 1229 (1964).

DHALIWAL, S. S.: Studies on histocompatibility mutations in mouse tumor cells using isogenic strains of mice. Genet. Res. 2, 309 (1961).

DIXON, F.: Immunopathology of the kidney. Symposium on immunopathology. Monte Carlo 1965.

ENGELL, H. C.: Cancer cells in the blood. Ann. Surg. 149, 457 (1959).

EVANS, C. A., and Y. ITO: Antitumor immunity in the Shope papilloma carcinoma complex of rabbits. J. nat. Cancer Inst. 36, 1161 (1966).

EVERSON, T. C., and W. H. COLE: Spontaneous regression of cancer: preliminary report. Ann. Surg. 144, 366 (1956).

FARDON, J. C., and E. PRINCE: An attempt to induce resistance in an inbred strain of mice by ligation of a homologous tumor. Cancer Res. 13, 19 (1953).

FINK, M. A., and V. QUINN: Antibody production in inbred strains of mice. J. Immunol. 70, 61 (1953).

—, P. SMITH, and M. F. ROTHLAUF: Antibody production in BALB/C mice following injection of lyophilized tumor S 621 in Freund's adjuvant. Proc. Soc. exp. Biol. Med. 90, 590 (1955).

—, G. D. SNELL, and D. KELTON: Demonstration of antibody in strain BALB/c mice to homologous tumour S 621 by the use of two technics: anaphylaxis and tumour regression. Cancer Res. 13, 666 (1953).

FINKELSTEIN, M. S., and J. W. UHR: Specific inhibition of antibody formation by passively administered 19 S and 7 S antibody. Science 146, 67 (1964).

FINNEY, J. W., and E. H. BRYER: Studies in tumor autoimmunity. Proc. Amer. Ass. Cancer Res. 3, 110 (1960).

— —, and R. H. WILSON: Studies in tumor autoimmunity. Cancer Res. 20, 351 (1960).

FISHER, B., and E. R. FISHER: Experimental evidence in support of the the dormant tumor cells. Science L30, 918 (1959).

FLEXNER, S., and J. W. JOBLING: Restraint in promotion of tumor growth. Proc. Soc. exp. Biol. Med. 5, 16 (1907).

— —, and M. L. MENTEN: Experimental studies on tumors. Monogr. Rockefeller Inst. Med. Res. 1910.

FOLEY, E. J.: Immunity of C3H mice to lymphosarcoma 6C3HED following regression of the transplanted tumor. Proc. Soc. exp. Biol. Med. 80, 131 (1952).

— Antigenic properties of methylcholantrene induced tumors in mice of the strain of origin. Cancer Res. 13, 835 (1953).

FRANKER, C. K., and J. J. QUILLIGAN: Genetic aspect of resistance to Friend leukemia virus. Proc. Soc. exp. Biol. Med. **121**, 1090 (1966).

GILDEN, R. V., R. I. CARP, F. TAGUCHI, and V. DEFENDI: The nature and localization of the SV 40 induced complement fixing antigen. Proc. nat. Acad. Sci. **53**, 684, 1965.

GINSBURG, H., and L. SACHS: Destruction of mouse and rat embryo cells in tissue culture by lymph node cells from unsensitized rats. Cell. comp. Physiol. **66**, 199 (1965).

GLOBERSON, A., and M. FELDMAN: Antigenic specificity of benzpyren induced sarcomas. J. nat. Cancer Inst. **32**, 1229 (1964).

GOLDIN, A., and S. R. HUMPHREYS: Studies of immunity in mice surviving systemic leukemia L 1210. J. nat. Cancer Inst. **24**, 283 (1960).

GOLDNER H., A. E. BODGEN, and P. M. APTEKMAN: Immunity against a transplantable ascites tumor of spontaneous origin in an inbred rat strain. J. Immunol. **82**, 520 (1959).

GORDON, J.: Isoantigenicity of liver tumors induced by an azodye. Brit. J. Cancer **19**, 387 (1965).

GORER, P. A.: Some recent work on tumor immunity. Adv. Cancer Research **4**, 149 (1956).

—, and O. B. AMOS: Passive immunity in mice against C57BL leukosis EL 4 by means of isoimmunine serum. Cancer Res. **16**, 338 (1956).

—, and N. KALISS: The effect of isoantibodies in vivo on three different transplanatbel neoplasms in mice. Cancer Res. **19**, 824 (1959).

— The antigenic structure of tumors. Adv. Immunol. **1**, 345 (1961).

—, and Z. B. MIKULSKA: The antibody response to tumor inoculation — improved method of antibody detection. Cancer Res. **14**, 651 (1954).

—, M. A. TUFFREY, and J. R. BATCHELOR: Serological studies on the X antigens. Ann. N. Y. Acad. Sci. **101**, 5 (1962).

GORODILOVA, V. V., I. G. SILNIYA, and Z. M. SARAYEVA: First experiment with vaccination against metastasis of breast carcinoma (in Russian). Vop. Onkol. **11**, 22 (1965).

GOWANS, J. L., J. D. McGREGOR, D. M. COWEN, and C. E. FORD: Initation of immune response by small lymphocytes. Nature **196**, 651 (1962).

GRACE, J. T.: Clinical aspects of immunity in untreated cancer. Ann. N. Y. Ac. Sci. **114**, 736 (1964).

—, and T. L. DAO: Etiology of inflammatory reaction in breast carcinoma. Surg. Forum **9**, 611 (1958).

—, and T. KONDO: Ivestigation of host resistance in cancer patient. Ann. Surg. **14**, 633 (1958).

—, D. M. PERESE, R. S. METZGAR, T. SASABE, and J. HOLDRIDGE: Tumor autograft responses in patient with gliobalstoma multiforme. J. Neurosurg. **18**, 159 (1961).

GRAFFI, A., G. PASTERNAK, and K. H. HORN: The intravenous mode of application for testing induced isoimmunity by tumors in mice. Acta biol. med. germ. **9**, 318 (1964).

GRAHAM, J. B.: The effect of vaccine in cancer patients. Surg. Gyn. Obstr. **109**, 131 (1959).

—, and R. M. GRAHAM: Antibodies elicited by cancer in patients. J. Amer. med. Ass. **8**, 409 (1955).

GROSS, L. A.: Intradermal immunisation of C3H mice against a sarcoma originated in animal of the same line. Cancer Res. **3**, 326 (1943).

— The importance of dosage in the intradermal immunisation against transplantable neoplasms. Cancer Res. **3**, 770 (1943).

HABEL, K.: Resistance of polyoma virus immune animals to transplanted polyoma tumors. Proc. Soc. exp. Biol. Med. **106**, 722 (1961).

— The relationship between polyoma virus multiplication, immunological competence and resistance to tumor challenge. Ann. N. Y. Acad. Sci. **101**, 173 (1962).

— Polyoma tumor antigen in cells transformed in vitro by polyoma virus. Virology **18**, 553 (1962).

— The relationship between polyoma virus multiplication, immunological competence and resistance to tumor challenge in the mouse. Ann. N. Y. Acad. Sci. **101**, 173 (1962).

—, and P. ATANASIUS: Transplantation of polyoma virus induced tumor in hamster. Proc. Soc. exp. Biol. Med. **102**, 99 (1959).

—, and B. F. EDDY: Specifity of resistance to tumour challenge of polyoma and SV 40 virus immune hamsters. Proc. Soc. exp. Biol. Med. **113**, 1 (1963).

HARE, J. D.: Transplant immunity to polyoma induced tumors: II. Evidence for host dependent immunogenic variation of polyoma virus. Proc. Soc. exp. Biol. Med. **117**, 598 (1964).

—, and H. R. MORGAN: A polyoma virus variant with a new antigenic determinant. Virology **19**, 105 (1963).

HARRIS, R. J. C., and P. SIMONS: In: Mechanism of immunological tolerance. Prague 1961.

— In: Specific tumor antigens. Muksngaard 1967.

HAUSCHKA, T. S.: Immunological aspects of cancer: a review. Cancer Res. **12**, 615 (1952).

HELLSTRÖM, K. E.: Studies on isoantigenic variation of mouse tumor cells in vitro. J. nat. Cancer Inst. **25**, 237 (1960).

—, and K. E. MÖLLER: Immunological and immunogenetic aspects of tumor transplantation. Progr. Allergy **9**, 158 (1965).

HIRSCH, H. M.: Tumor isoimmunity. Experientia **14**, 269, 1958.

—, J. J. BITTNER, H. COLE, and I. IVERSEN: Can the inbred mouse be immunised against its own tumor. Cancer Res. **18**, 344 (1958).

—, and J. IVERSEN: Accelerated development of spontaneous mammary tumors in mice pretreated with mammary tumor tissue and adjuvant. Cancer Res. **21**, 752 (1961).

HIRST, A. E., and R. T. BERGMAN: Carcinoma of the prostate in men 80 or more years old. Cancer **7**, 136 (1954).

HOLM, G., and D. PERLMANN: Phytomaemagglutinin induced cytotoxic action of unsenstized immunological competent cells on allogenic and xenogenic tissue culture cells. Nature **207**, 818 (1965).

— —, and B. WERNER: Phytohaemagglutinin induced cytotoxic action of normal lymphoid cells on cells in tissue culture. Nature **203**, 841 (1964).

HORN, K. H., G. PASTERNAK, und A. GRAFFI: Versuche zur Induktion von Immunität gegen methylcholantrene Tumoren durch Vorbehandlung der Mäuse mit homologen und heterologen Tumortransplantaten. Acta. biol. med. germ. **9**, 309 (1962).

HOUGHTON, G.: Extraction of H-2 antigen from mouse tumor cells. Transplantation **2**, 251 (1964).

— Moloney virus induced leukemia of mice: measurement in vitro of specific antigen. Science **147**, 506 (1965).

HUEBNER, R. J., R. M. CHANOCH, B. A. RUBIN, and M. J. CASEY: Induction by adenovirus type 7 of tumors in hamsters having the antigenic characteristic of SV 40 virus. Proc. nat. Ac. Sci. **52**, 1333 (1964).

HUGHES, L. E., and B. LYTTON: Antigenic properties of human tumors: delayed cutaneous hypersensitivity reaction. Brit. med. J. **1**, 209 (1964).

ISHIBASHI, Y.: The effect of bobe marrow transplantation on the survival of tumor bearing patients and animals. Japan J. exp. Med. **35**, 419 (1965).

ISOJIMA, S., R. M. GRAHAM, and J. B. GRAHAM: Sterility in female guinea pigs induce by injection with testis Science **129**, 44 (1959).

ITOH, T., and C. M. SOUTHAM: Isoantibodies to human cancer cells in cancer patients following cancer homotransplant. J. Immunol. **93**, 926 (1964).

JAKKOLA, M.: Inherotance of resistance to polyoma tumorgenesis in mice. J. nat. Cancer Inst. **35**, 595 (1965).

JAKOUBKOVÁ, J.: The role of immunity in the antitumor reactions in clinical practice. Neoplasma **12**, 131 (1965).

—, V. BEK, N. HAVRÁNKOVÁ, L. PALEČEK, and P. KOLDOVSKÝ: Fate of lung metastasis of hypernephroma (Grawitz tumor) (in Czech). Čs. radiol. **19**, 393 (1965).

—, P. KOLDOVSKÝ, V. BEK, A. MÁJSKÝ, V. SCHNEID, and M. VOPATOVÁ: To the problem of immunotherapy of choriocarcinoma. Neoplasma **12**, 531 (1965).

JONSSON, N.: Studies on the occurence of common specific transplantation antigen in Rous tumors of various mammalian species. Acta path. microbiol. scand. **67**, 339 (1966).

—, and H. O. SJÖGREN: Isograft resistance to Rous sarcoma in mice inoculated with Rous chicken sarcoma when newborn. Exp. Cell Res. **40**, 159 (1965).

— — Specific transplantation immunity in relation to Rous sarcoma virus tumorigenesis in mice. J. exp. Med. **123**, 487 (1966).

JURAND, J., and R. HIRAMOTO: Antigenic relationship of mouse rhabdomyosarcoma to human rhabdomyosarcoma and to human and mouse muscel. Cancer Res. **26**, 1486 (1966).

KALISS, N.: Imunological enhencement and inhibition of tumor growth: relationship to various immunological mechanisms. Fed. Proc. **24**, 1024 (1965).

—, and L. BRYANT: Immunological enhencement. J. Nat. Cancer Inst. **20**, 691 (1958).

—, and O. NEWTON: The effect of injection dosage level of lyophilized mouse tissue on the subsequent of tumor homiotransplants in mice. Cancer Res. **11**, 122 (1951).

—, and D. SPAIN: The effect of the prior injection of lyophilized mouse tissue on the survival of normal tissue homografts in mice. Cancer Res. **12**, 272 (1952).

KANDUTSCH, A. A.: Intracellular distribution and extraction of tumor homograft enhencing antigens. Cancer Res. **20**, 264 (1960).

KELOFF, G., and P. K. VOGT: Localization of avian tumor virus group specific antigen in cell and virus. Virology **29**, 377 (1966).

KHERRA, K. S., A. ASHKENAZI, F. RAPP, and J. L. MELNICK: Immunity in hamsters to cell transformed in vitro and in vivo by SV 40. J. Immunol. **91**, 604 (1963).

KIDD, J. G.: The course of virus induced rabbit pappilomas as determined by virus, cells and host. J. exp. Med. **67**, 551 (1938).

KIDD, J.: Suppressio of the growth of Brown Pearce tumor cells by a specific antibody, with a consideration on the nature of the reacting cell constituent. J. exp. Med. **83**, 227 (1946).

KIRSCHSTEIN, R. L., A. S. RABSON, and E. A. PETERES: Oncogenic activity of adenovirus 12 in thymectomized BALB/c and C3H/HeN mice. Proc. Soc. Exp. biol. med. **117**, 198 (1964).

KLEIN, E.: Isoantigenicity of X-ray inactovated implants of homotransplantable and non-homotransplantable mouse sarcoma. Transpl. Bull. **6**, 420 (1959).

—, and G. KLEIN: Mechanism of induced change in transplantation specificy of a mouse tumor passed through hybrid hosts. Transpl. Bull. **2**, 136 (1956).

— — Antigenic properties of lymphomas induced by Moloney agent. J. Nat. Cancer Inst. **32**, 547 (1964).

— — Antibody response and leukemic development in mice inoculated neonatally with the Moloney virus.. Cancer Res. **25**, 851 (1965).

— — Immunological tolerance of neonatally infected mice to Moloney leukemia virus. Nature **209**, 163 (1966).

—, and L. REVESZ: Permanent modification (mutation?) of a histocompatibility gene in a heterogenous tumor. J. nat. Cancer Inst. **19**, 95 (1957).

—, and H. O. SJÖGREN: Studies on the effect of iso-antiserum on mouse sarcoma cells. Transpl. Bull. **26**, 442 (1960 a).

— — Humoral and cellular factors in homograft a and isograft immunity against sarcoma cells. Cancer Res. **20**, 452 (1960 b).

KLEIN, G., H. O. SJÖGREN, and E. KLEIN: Demonstration of host resistance against isotransplants of lymphomas induced by the Gross agent. Cancer Res. **22**, 955 (1962).

— — — Demonstration of host resistance against sarcomas induce by implantation of cellophane films in isologous (syngeneic) recipient. Cancer Res. **23**, 84 (1963).

—, P. CLIFFORD, E. KLEIN, and J. STJERNSWÄRD: Search for tumor specific immune reaction in Burkitt lymphoma patients by the membrane immunofluorescence reaction. Proc. Nat. Ac. Sci. **55**, 1628 (1966).

—, H. O. SJÖGREN, E. KLEIN, and K. E. HELLSTRÖM: Demonstration of resistance against methylcholantrene induce sarcomas in the primary autochtonous host. Cancer Res. **20**, 1561 (1960).

KLEMENT, V.: Pathogenicity of Rous virus for adult rats. Folia Biol. **11**, 438 (1965).

KOCH, M. A., and A. B. SABIN: Specifity of virus induced resistance to transplantation of polyoma and SV 40 tumors in adult hamsters. Proc. Soc. Exp. Biol. Med. **113**, 4 (1963).

KOIKE, A., G. E. MOOR, C. B. MENDOZA, and A. L. WATNE: Heterologous, homologous and autologous transplantation of human tumors. Cancer **16**, 716 (1963).

KOLDOVSKÝ, P.: The question of the choice of method to induce anti-tumour isoimmunity within a group of mice with controlled antigenic homogeneity. Folia Biol. (Praha) **7**, 115 (1961).

— Passive tranfer of anti-tumour isoimmunity. Folia Biol. (Praha) **7**, 157 (1961).

KOLDOVSKÝ, P.: The question of the universality of tumor antigen in isologous and homologous relatioships. Ibid. **7**, 162 (1961).
— Isoimmunity against an induced primary tumor. Ibid. **7**, 170 (1961).
— Failure to induce isoimmunity against leukemia induced by irradiation in strain CBA mice. Ibid. **8**, 360 (1962).
— Specific tumour immunity and its use in immunotherapy of experimental tumor. Acta U.I.C.C. **18**, 87 (1962).
— The antigenic specifity of tumours induce in mice by the Rous sarcoma virus. Neoplasma **12**, 155 (1965).
— Immunity against tumour tissue. Neoplasma **12**, 113 (1965).
— An attempt at in vitro sensitization of immunologically competent cells against tumour specific antigen. Folia biol. (Praha) **12**, 238 (1966).
— Annual report of Imperial Cancer Research Fund 1966.
— On the role of cells and sear in specific antitumor reaction. In Specific Tumor Antigen. Symposium of the U.I.C.C. Munksgaard 1967.
—, and J. BUBENÍK: Difference between the parental strain and the F_1 hybrid in the isoimmune reaction to tumours. Folia Biol. (Praha) **9**, 420 (1963).
— — Occurence of tumors in mice after inoculation of Rous sarcoma and antigenic changes in these tumors. Folia Biol. **10**, 81 (1964).
— — Resistance to RSV induce tumours in mice. Folia Biol. (Praha) **11**, 198 (1965).
— — The effect of immunity against sex antigen on tumour graft containing sex antigen. Folia Biol. (Praha) **11**, 266 (1965).
— — Specific antigen of tumours induced by Rous sarcoma in inbred mice. Proc. Symp. Mutational Process Prague, 331 (1965).
—, and A. LENEGEROVÁ: A combination of specific antitumour therapy and x ray irradiation. Folia Biol. (Praha) **6**, 441 (1960).
—, and J. SVOBODA: Induction of tolerance to tumour antigen mechanism of immunological tolerance. Prague 1962, pp. 215.
— — On the question of the mechanism of growth of a tumour against isoimmunity. Folia Biol. (Praha) **8**, 95 (1962).
— — On the question of the role of heterologous tolerance in possibility to immunize against tumour antigen. Folia Biol. (Praha) **8**, 101 (1962).
— — Sensitivity of a tumour to immunity in relationship to its antigenicity. Folia Biol. (Praha) **8**, 144 (1962).
— — Cross reaction between benzpyrene induced tumors in rats and mice. Folia Biol. (Praha) **9**, 233 (1963).
— — Induction of tumours by Rous sarcoma virus in adult mice. Folia Biol. (Praha) **11**, 203 (1965).
— —, and J. BUBENÍK: Further studies in the immunobiology of tumour RVA 2 induced by RSV in C57BL strain mice. Folia Biol. (Praha) **12**, 1 (1966).
KOPROWSKI, H., and M. V. FERNANDES: Autosensitisation reaction in vitro. J. exp. Med. **116**, 467 (1962).
—, G. THEIS, and R. LOVE: Immunological tolerance in tumor studies. Adaptation of ascites tumor to homologous and heterologous host. Proc. roy. Soc. Ser. B. **146**, 37 (1956).
LAICOPOULUS, P., and J. H. GOOD: Transplantation tolerance induced in adult mice by protein overloding of donors. Science **146**, 1305 (1964).
LAVRIN, D. H., P. B. BLAIR, and D. W. WEIS: Immunology of spontaneous mammary carcinoma in mice. III. Immunogenicity of C3H preneoplastic hyperplastic alveolar nodules in C3H/f hosts. Cancer Res. **26**, 293 (1966).
— — — Immunology of spontaneous mammary carcinomas in mice. IV. Association of the mammary tumor virus with the immunogenicity of C3H nodules and tumors. Cancer Res. **26**, 929 (1966).
LAW, L. W.: Genetic studies in experimental cancer. Adv. Cancer Res. **2**, 281 (1954).
— Immunological responsivness and the induction of experimental neoplasms. Cancer Res. **26**, 1121 (1966).
LEWIS, M. R., and P. M. APTEKMAN: Antigenicity of sarcomata undergoing atrophy in rats. J. Immunol. **67**, 193 (1951).

Líbánský, J.: Study of immunological reactivity in haemoblastosis, circulating antibody formation and responsivness to antigenic stimulus in leukemia, malignant lymphoma and myeloblastosis. Blood **25**, 169 (1965).

Lindner, O. E. A.: Survival of skin homografts in methylcholantrene treated mice and in mice with spontaneous mammary cancer. Cancer Res. **22**, 380 (1962).

—, and E. Klein: Skin and tumor grafting in co-isogenic lines of mice and their hybrids. J. Nat. Cancer Inst. **24**, 707 (1960).

Little, C. C., and E. E. Tyzzer: Further experimental studies on the inheritance and susceptibility to transplantable tumour, carcinoma of the Japanese Waltzing mouse. J. med. Res. **33**, 393 (1916).

Lumsden, T.: Tumor immunity. Amer. J. Cancer **15**, 563 (1931).

Maisin, J. H. F.: Essaiy d'immunoprophylaxie du cancer experimental. Acat. U.I.C.C. **19**, 94 (1963).

— Role of thymus and thymus factor in the induction of 20-methylcholantrene skin cancer in mice. Nature **202**, 202 (1964).

Makari, J. G., and T. Hayton: The tumor skin test: a five year follow up study. Trans. N. Y. Ac. Sci. ser. II. **28**, 198 (1965).

Malmgren, R. A., B. F. Bennison, and T. W. McKinley: Reduced antibody titers in mice treated with carcinogenic and cancer chemotherapeutic agents. Pros. Soc. exp. Biol. Med. **79**, 484 (1952).

—, A. S. Rabson, and P. H. Carney: Immunity and viral carcinogenesis. Effect of thymectomy on polyoma virus carcinogenesis in mice. J. nat. Cancer. Inst. **33**, 101 (1964).

Martinez, C.: Effect of early thymectomy on the development of mammary tumors in mice. Nature **203**, 1188 (1964).

—, J. B. Aust, J. J. Bittner, and R. Good: Continuous growth of isotransplants of mammary tumor associated with development of immunity in mice. Cancer Res. **18**, 344 (1958).

—, H. Kelman, and R. A. Good: Transplantability changes of mouse mammary tumors after passage through tolerant homologous recipients. Proc. Soc. exp. Biol. Med. **104**, 413 (1960).

Mathé, G., J. Dausset, E. Hervet, J. L. Amiel, J. Colombani, and G. Brule: Immunological studies in patients with placental choriocarcinoma. J. nat. Cancer Inst. **33**, 193 (1964).

Matsuomoto, T.: Immunological studies of tumour. III: Effect of homologous antiserum on Yoshida sarcoma cells in vivo. Cytologia **25**, 86 (1965).

—, K. Otsu, and T. Komeda: Induction of host resistance against isotransplantation of C-1498 leukemia by spleen cells from tumour bearing donors. Gann **57**, 143 (1966).

Matsuoha, Y., M. Nakayama, T. Hamaoka, Y. Okada, and Y. Yamamura: Antibody response of the tumor bearing animals. Gann **56**, 503 (1965).

McKhann, C. F.: Weak histocompatibility genes: the effect of dose and pretreatment of immunizing cells. J. Immunol. **88**, 500 (1962).

— The effect of x-ray on the antigenicity of donor cells in transplantation immunity. J. Immunol. **92**, 811 (1964).

— Methods of detecting cancer antigens and antitumor antibody. Fed. Proc. **24**, 1033 (1965).

Medawar, P. B., and E. M. Sparrow: The effect of adenocorticotrophic hormone and pregnancy on skin transplantation immunnity in mice. J. Endocrinol. **14**, 240 (1956).

Miller, J. F. A. P., G. A. Grant, and F. J. C. Roe: Effecto- of thymectomy on the induction of skin tumors by 3,4-benzopyrene. Nature **199**, 920 (1963).

Miroff, G. C., C. Martinez, and J. J. Bittner: Acceleration in transplantation and killing time of mammary tumors in mice pretreated with heat stable tumor tissue preparation. Cancer Res. **15**, 347 (1955).

Mitchison, N. A.: Studies on the immunological response to foreign tumor transplantation in the mouse. I: The role of lymphnode cells in conferring immunity by adoptive transfer. J. exp. Med. **102**, 157 (1955).

Möller, E.: Antagostic effect of humoral antibodies on the in vitro cytotoxicity of immune lymphoid cells. J. exp. Med. **122**, 11 (1965).

MöLLER, E.: Isoantigenic properties of tumors transgressing histocompatibility barriers of the H-2 systems. J. nat. Cancer Inst. 33, 979 (1964).

MöLLER, G.: Demonstration of mouse isoantigens on the cellular level by the fluorescen antibody technique. J. Exp. med. 114, 415 (1961).

— Studies on the mechanism of immunological enhencement. I: Specifity of immunological enhencement. J. nat. Cancer Inst. 30, 1153 (1963). — II: Effect of isoantibodies on various tumor cells. Folia Biol. (Praha) 20, 1177 (1963). — III: Interaction between humoral isoantibodies and immune lymphnode cells. J. nat. Cancer Inst. 30, 1205 (1963).

— Effect of tumor growth in syngenic recipients of antibodies against tumor specific antigens of methylcholantrene induced sarcomas. Nature 204, 846 (1964).

MOLOMUT, N.: Host induced alteration in strain specifity of Sarcoma I in mice. Reversibility of the change. Cancer Res. 18, 906 (1958).

—, and L. W. SMITH: Host induce alteration in strain specifity of Sarcoma I in mice. Effect of active immunisation of the host. Cancer Res. 17, 92 (1957).

MORI, R., K. NOMOTO, G. KIMURA, and K. TAKEYA: Effect of thymectomy on polyoma induction in CF_1 mice. Arch. ges. Virusforsch. 17, 186 (1966).

NUNGESTER, V. J., and H. FISHER: The inactivation in vivo of mouse lymphosarcoma 6C3HED by antibodies produced in a foreign host species. Cancer Res. 14, 284 (1954).

OLD, L. J., and D. A. CLARENCE: Effect of BCG infection on transplanted tumors in the mouse. Nature 184, 291 (1959).

—, E. A. BOYSE, D. A. CLARKE, and E. CARSWELL: Antigenic properties of chemically induced tumors. Ann. N. Y. Acad. Sci. 101, 80 (1962).

— —, and F. LILLY: Formation of cytotoxic antibody against leukemias induce by Friend virus. Cancer Res. 23, 1063 (1963).

— — —, and N. LUELL: Antigenic properties of experimental leukemias. II: Immunological studies in vivo with C57BL/6 radiation induce leukemia. J. nat. Cancer Inst. 31, 987 (1963).

— —, and E. STOCKERT: Antigenic properties of experimental leukemias. I: Serological studies in vitro with spontaneous and radiation induced leukemias. J. nat. Cancer Inst. 31, 977 (1963).

OPPENHEIMER, B. J., E. T. OPPENHEIMER, F. R. EIROCH, I. DARISHEVSKY, and A. P. STOUT: Further studies of polymers as carcinogens in animals. Cancer Res. 15, 333 (1955).

ORAVEC, C.: Interaction of properdin system with tumorous cells. Neoplasma 11, 47 (1964).

PARROT, D.: Annual Report of Imperial Cancer Research Fund 1965.

PASTERNAK, G., A. GRAFFI u. K. II. HORN: Der Nachweis individual spezifischer Antigenität bei UV induzierten Sarkomen der Maus. Acta biol. med. germ. 13, 276 (1964).

—, A. GRAFFI, F. HOFFMAN, and K. H. HORN: Demonstration of resistance against carcinomas of the skin induced by dimethylbenzanthracene in mice of the strain XVII/Blr. Nature.

—, K. H. HORN u. A. GRAFFI: Immunologische Cross-Versuche mit Methclontrentumoren eines Mäuseinzuchtstammes. Folia Biol. (Praha) 9, 306 (1962).

—, and L. PASTERNAK: Demonstration of Graffi leukemic virus and virus induced antigens in leukemic and nonleukemic tissue of mice. J. nat. Cancer Inst. 38, 157 (1967).

PAYNE, F. E., J. J. SOLOMON, and H. G. PURCHASE: Immunofluorescent studies of group specific antigen of the avian sarcoma-leukosis viruses. Proc. nat. Acad. Sci. (Wash.) 55, 341 (1966).

PELNER, L.: Host tumor antagonism XXXIII. Cancer immunity: a review and an analysis of some factors in host resistance to cancer. J. Amer. geriat. Soc. 11, 843 (1963).

POOL, E. H., and G. R. DUNLAP: Cancer cells in blood stream. Am. C. Cancer 21, 99 (1934).

PREHN, R. T.: Tumor specific immunity to transplanted dibenzanthracene sarcomas. Cancer Res. 20, 1614 (1960).

— Specific homograft tolerance induced by successive matings and implications concrening choriocarcinoma. J. nat. Cancer Inst. 25, 883 (1960).

— Failure of immunisation against tumorigenesis. J. nat. Cancer Inst. 26, 223 (1961).

— Function of depressed immunologic reactivity during carcinogenesis. J. nat. Cancer Inst. 31, 791 (1963).

— Cancer antigens in tumors induced by chemicals. Fed. Proc. 24, 1018 (1965).

PREHN, R. T., and J. M. MAIN: Immunity to methylcholantrene induced sarcomas. J. nat. Cancer. Inst. 18, 769 (1957).

PRINCE, J. E., J. C. FARDON, L. G. NUTINI, and G. S. SPERTI: Induced resistance to an indigenous transplantable mouse tumor. Cancer Res. 17, 312 (1957).

RADZICHOVSKAJA, R.: Specific resistance to tumors of virus origin (in Russian). Vop. Sovr. Biol. 62, 274 (1966).

RAPP, F., S. BUTTELM, and J. L. MELNICK: Viru induced intranuclear antigen in cells transformed by papova virus SV 40. Proc. Soc. exp. Biol. Med. 116, 1131 (1964).

REVESZ, L.: Detection of antigenic differences in isologous host tumor systems by pretreatment with heavily irradiated tumor cells. Cancer Res. 20, 443 (1960).

ROBINSON, E., and A. HOCHMAN: Comparative study on the lymphocytes transfer test with lymphocytes from normal donors and cancer patients. J. nat. Cancer Inst. 36, 819 (1966).

—, J. SHULMAN, N. BEN-HUR, H. ZUCKERMAN, and Z. NEUMAN: Immuno logical studies and behaviour of husband and foreign homografts with chorionepthelioma. Lancet 300 (1963).

ROSENAU, W., and H. D. MOON: Lysis of homologous cells by sensitized lymphocytes in tissue culture. J. nat. Cancer Inst. 27, 471 (1961).

— — Cellular reaction to methylcholantrene induced sarcomas transplanted to isogenic mice. Lab. Inv. 15, 1212 (1966).

RUBIN, B. A.: Cancerogen induced tolerance to homotransplantation of normal tissue. Proc. Amer. Ass. Cancer Res. 3, 146 (1960).

RUBIN, H., L. FANSHIER, A. CORNELIUS, and W. F. HUGHES: Tolerance and immunity in chickens after congenital and contact infection with avian leukosis virus. Virology 17, 143 (1962).

SACHS, L., and D. MEDINA: Polyoma virus mutant with a reduction in tumor formation. Nature 187, 715 (1960).

— Tumor transplantation in mice inoculated with polyoma virus. Exp. Cell Res. 24, 185 (1961).

— The transplantability of an x-ray and virus induced leukemia in isologous mice inoculated with a leukemia virus. J. nat. Cancer Inst. 29, 759 (1962).

SANFORD, K. K., G. G. LIKELY, and W. R. EARLE: The development of variation in transplantability and morphology within a clone of mouse fibroblasts transformed to sarcoma producing cells in vitro. J. nat. Cancer Inst. 15, 215 (1954).

—, G. L. HOBBS, and W. E. EARLE: The tumor producing capacity of strain L mouse cells after 10 years in vitro. Cancer Res. 16, 162 (1956).

—, R. M. MERWIN, G. L. HOBBS, M. C. FIORAMONT, and W. R. EARLE: Studies on the difference in sarcoma producing capacity of two lines of mouse cells derived in vitro from one cells. J. nat. Cancer Inst. 20, 121 (1958).

SCHMAUCH, G.: Das syncioma malignum vaginale p. p. mature ohne Geschwulstbildung im Uterus und seine Ätiologie. Z. Geburtsh. Gynäkol. 49, 387 (1903).

SCHWARTZ, E. E., and S. WINSTEIN: Serum properdin in tumor-bearing mice. II. The influence of tumors of different origin. Cancer Res. 24, 830 (1964).

SCHWARTZ, ST. O., and S. SCHOLMAN: The passive immunisation of C3H mice against the induction of leukemia. Proc. Am. Ass. Cancer Res. 2, 344 (1958).

SJÖGREN, H. O.: Transplantation method as a toll for detection of tumor specific antigens. Progr. exp. Tumor Research 6, 289 (1964).

— Studies the specific transplantation resistance against polyoma virus induced tumor. I: Transplantation resistance induced by polyoma infection. J. nat. Cancer Inst. 32, 361 (1962). — II: Studies of the mechanism of the resistance induced by polyoma infection. J. nat. Cancer Inst. 32, 375 (1964). — III: Transplantation resistance against genetically compatible polyoma tumors induced by polyoma tumor homografts. J. nat. Cancer Inst. 32, 645 (1964). — IV: Stability of the polyoma antigen. J. nat. Cancer Inst. 32, 661 (1964).

— In: Tumour specific antigens. Kopenhagen: Munksgaard 1967.

—, and I. HELLSTRÖM: In vivo and in vitro demonstration of the polyoma specific antigen induced in polyoma infected Moloney lymphoma cells. In: Tumour specific antigens. Munksgaard 1967, pp. 163.

SjöGREN, H. O., I. HELLSTRÖM, and G. KLEIN: Resistance of polyoma virus immunized mice against transplantation of established polyoma tumors. Exp. Cell Research **23**, 204 (1961).

—, and N. JONSSON: Resistance against transplantation of mouse tumors induced by Rous sarcoma virus. Exp. Cell. Res. **32**, 618 (1963).

—, and N. RINGERTZ: Histopathology and transplantability of polyoma induced tumors in strain A/sn and their coisogenic resistant (IR) sublines. J. nat. Cancer Inst. **28**, 85 (1962).

SLETTENMARK, B., and E. KLEIN: Cytotoxic and neutralization tests with serum and lymph-node cells of isologous mice with induced resistance against Gross lymphoma. Cancer Res. **22**, 947 (1962).

SMITH, J. L., and J. S. STEHLIN: Spontaneous regression of primary malignant melanomas with regional metastases. Cancer **18**, 1399 (1965).

SMITH, R. R., L. THOMAS, and A. W. HILBERG: Cancer cell contamination in operation wounds. Cancer **11**, 53 (1958).

SMITHERS, D. W.: Spontaneous regression of tumours. Clinical Radiol. **13**, 132 (1962).

SNELL, G. D., J. H. WINN, J. H. STIMPFLING, and S. J. PARKET: Depression by antibody of the immune response to homografts and its role in immunological enhencement. J. exp. Med. **112**, 293 (1960).

SOUTHAM, C. M.: Evidence of immunological reactions to autochtonous cancer in men. Europ. J. Cancer **1**, 173 (1965).

SPJUT, H. J.: Cancer cells in pleural cavity washing. Cancer **11**, 1222 (1958).

STEINER, P. E., S. N. MAIMOR, W. L. PARKER, and J. B. KIRSNER: Gastric cancer: morphologic factors in five years survival after gastrectomy. Amer. J. Path. **24**, 947 (1948).

STERN, K.: A new approach to tumour immunity. Nature **183**, 787 (1960).

STJERNSWÄRD, J.: Effect of noncarcinogenic and carcinogenic hydrocarbons an antibody-forming cells measured at the celluar level in vitro. J. nat. Cancer Inst. **36**, 1189 (1966).

— Immunidepressive effect of 3-methylcholantrene antibody formation at the cellular level and reaction against weak antigenic homografts. J. nat. Cancer Inst. **35**, 885 (1962).

STRONG, L. C.: A genetic analysis of the factors underlying susceptibility to transplantable tumors. J. exp. Zool. **36**, 671 (1922).

— On the occurence of mutations within transplantable neoplasms. Genetics **11**, 294 (1926).

— Transplantation studies on tumor arising spontaneously in heterozygous individuals. I: Experimental evidence for the theory that tumor cell has derived from a definitive somatic cell by process analogous to somatic mutation. J. Cancer Res. **13**, 103 (1929).

— Genetic concept for the origin of cancer. Historical review. Ann. N. Y. Acad. Sci. **71**, 810 (1958).

SVOBODA, J.: Aspects of tolerance to Rous virus. In: Mechanism of immunological tolerance. Prague 1961.

TELLER, M., G. W. STOKER, M. CURLETT, D. KULISEK, and D. CURTIS: Aging and cancerogenesis. J. nat. Cancer Inst. **33**, 649 (1964).

TER-GRIGOROV, V. S., and J. S. IRLIN: Suppression of resistance of mice to the polyoma virus connected with lymphatic tissue destruction following injection of tissue extracts from sheep suffering from pulmonary adematosis. Neoplasma **11**, 27 (1964).

TEVETHIA, S. S., and F. RAPP: Demonstration of new surface antigen in cells transformed by papovirus SV 40 by cytotoxic tests. Proc. Soc. exp. Biol. Med. **120**, 455 (1965).

TOOLLAN, H. W.: Permanantly transplanted human tumors. Cancer Res. **17**, 418 (1957).

VANDEPUTTE, M., P. DENYS, R. LEYTEN, and P. DESOMER: The oncogenic activity of the polyoma virus in thymectomized rats. Life Sci. **7**, 475 (1963).

—, and P. DESOMER: Runting syndrome in mice inoculated with polyoma virus. J. nat. Cancer Inst. **35**, 237 (1965).

VREDOVOE, D. L., and W. H. HILDEMANN: Circulating small lymphocytes — immunologically competent cells with limited reactivities. Science **141**, 1272 (1963).

WAHREN, B.: Demonstration of a tumor specific antigen in spontaneously developing AKR leukemia. Int. J. Cancer **1**, 41 (1966).

— Cytotoxic assay and other immunological studies of leukemias induced by Friend virus. J. nat. Cancer Inst. **31**, 411 (1963).

WANG LIN-FANG, and LIANG CHIH-CHUAN: The effect of ionizing radiation in the antigenicity of bovine plasma albumin. Science Record 4, 404 (1960).

WATME, A. L., G. E. MOORE, and I. HATIBOGLU: Cancer cell in thoracic duct lymph. Proc. Am. Ass. Cancer Res. 3, 72 (1959).

WEISS, D. V., L. J. FAULKIN, and K. B. DEOME: Acquisition of hightened resistance and susceptibility to spontaneous mouse mammary carcinomas in the original host. Cancer Res. 24, 732 (1964).

WEISS, D., D. H. LAVRIN, M. DEZFULIAN, J. VAAGE, and P. B. BLAIR: Studies on the immunology of spontaneous mammary carcinoma in mice. UICC Monograph series vol. 2. Specific tumor antigens. Munksgaard 1966, p. 210.

WILSON, R. H., L. R. DEALNEY, V. JUREVICS, and A. SCHRAM: Immunochemical effect of prolonged exposure to the cancerogen 3-methylcholantrene. Cancer 19, 137 (1966).

WIMER, B. M.: Immunological aspects of cancer. Lancet II, 447 (1965).

WITEBSKI, E., N. R. ROSE, J. R. PAINE, and R. W. EGAN: Thyroid specific autoantibodies in immunology and cancer. Ann. N. Y. Acad. Sci. 69, 669 (1957).

WOGLOM, W. H.: Immunity to transplantable tumors. Cancer Rev. 4, 129 (1929).

WOODRUFF, M. F. A.: Transplantation immunity and the immunological problem of pregnancy. Proc. Roy. Soc., London, ser. B. 148, 68 (1957).

— Transplantation immunity and the immunological problem of pregnancy. Proc. Roy. Soc. B, 148 (1957).

—, and J. L. BOAK: Inhibition effect of preimmunized CBA spleen cells on transplants of A strain mouse mammary carcinoma in (CBA×A)F$_1$ hybrid recipients. Brit. J. Cancer 19, 411 (1965).

—, and B. NOLAN: Preliminary observations on treatment of advanced cancer by injection of allogeneic spleen cells. Lancet II, 426 (1963).

—, and M. SYMES: Evidence of loss of tumor specific antigen on repeatedly transplanting a tumor in the strain of origin. Brit. J. Cancer 16, 484 (1962).

— — The significance of splenomegaly in tumor bearing mice. Brit. J. Cancer 16, 120 (1962).

—, and M. O. SYMES: Evidence of loss of specific tumour antigen on repeatedly transplanting a tumour in the strain of origin. Brit. J. Cancer 16, 484 (1962).

YAMAGUCHI, I., T. TAKAHASHI, T. NARISAWA, and T. HIROKI: An experimental study on the effect of reticuloendothelial activity on metastases and reccurence of tumor. Tohoku J. exp. Med. 87, 338 (1965).

YOHN, D. S., C. A. FUNK, V. I. KALNINS, and J. T. GRACE: Sex related resistance in hamsters to adenovirus 12 oncogenesis. Influence of thymectomy in 3 weeks of age. J. nat. Cancer Inst. 35, 617 (1965).

YOON, L.: Eosinophiles and gastrointestinal cancer. Am. J. Surg. 97, 195 (1959).

ZEIDMAN, I., and I. M. BUSS: Experimental studies on the spread of cancer in the lymphatic system. I: Effectivness of the lymphnodes as barrier to the passage of embolic tumor cells. Cancer Res. 14, 403 (1954).

ZILBER, L. A.: Studies on tumor antigens. J. nat. Cancer Inst. 18, 341 (1957).

— Specific tumor antigens. Adv. Cancer Res. 6, 291 (1958).

—, and G. I. ABELEV: Virusologia i imunologija raka (in Russian). Moskva 1962.

—, and G. I. ABELEV: Virology and immunology of the cancer (in Russian). Moskva 1962.

Subject Index

Monographs already Published

In Production

In Preparation

ACKERMANN, N. B., Boston: Use of Radioisotopic Agents in the Diagnosis of Cancer

Asparaginase. Edited by E. GRUNDMANN, Wuppertal-Elberfeld, and OETTGEN, New York (Symposium)

BOIRON, M., Paris: The Viruses of the Leukemia-sarcoma Complex

CAVALIERE, R., A. ROSSI-FANELLI, B. MONDOVI, and G. MORICCA, Roma: Selective Heat Sensitivity of Cancer Cells

CHIAPPA, S., Milano: Endolymphatic Radiotherapy in Malignant Lymphomas

Cutane paraneoplastische Syndrome. Edited by J. J. HERZBERG, Bremen (Symposium)

DENOIX, P., Villejuif: Le traitement des cancers du sein

GRUNDMANN, E., Wuppertal-Elberfeld: Morphologie und Cytochemie der Carcinogenese

IRLIN, I. S., Moskva: Mechanisms of Viral Carcinogenesis

LANGLEY, F. A., and A. C. CROMPTON, Manchester: Epithelial Abnormalities of the Cervix Uteri

MATHÉ, G., Villejuif: L'Immunotherapie des Cancers

MEEK, E. S., Bristol: Antitumour and Antiviral Substances of Natural Origin

NEWMAN, M. K., Detroit: Neuropathies and Myopathies Associated with Occult Malignancies

OGAWA, K., Osaka: Ultrastructural Enzyme Cytochemistry of Azo-dye Carcinogenesis

PARKER, J. W., and R. J. LUKES, Los Angeles: Lymphocyte Transformation

PENN, I., Denver: Malignant Lymphomas in Transplant Patients

Recent Advances in the Treatment of Acute Leukemias. Edited by G. MATHÉ (Symposium)

SUGIMURA, T., Tokyo, H. ENDO, Fukuoka, and T. ONO, Tokyo: Chemistry and Biological Action of 4-Nitroquinoline 1-oxide, a Carcinogen

SZYMENDERA, J., Warsaw: The Metabolism of Bone Mineral in Malignancy

WEIL, R., Lausanne: Biological and Structural Properties of Polyoma Virus and its DNA

WILLIAMS, D. C., Caterham, Surrey: The Basis for Therapy of Hormon Sensitive Tumours

WILLIAMS, D. C., Caterham, Surrey: The Biochemistry of Metastasis

GPSR Compliance
The European Union's (EU) General Product Safety Regulation (GPSR) is a set
of rules that requires consumer products to be safe and our obligations to
ensure this.

If you have any concerns about our products, you can contact us on

ProductSafety@springernature.com

In case Publisher is established outside the EU, the EU authorized
representative is:

Springer Nature Customer Service Center GmbH
Europaplatz 3
69115 Heidelberg, Germany

www.ingramcontent.com/pod-product-compliance
Ingram Content Group UK Ltd.
Pitfield, Milton Keynes, MK11 3LW, UK
UKHW051346100726
473059UK00015B/2667